5.90

The Respiratory System

R. Grenville-Mathers MA, MD, FRCP

Consultant Physician,
Northwick Park Hospital and Critical Research Centre, Harrow
Edgware General Hospital,
Colindale Hospital and
Harrow Chest Clinic.

CHURCHILL LIVINGSTONE
EDINBURGH LONDON MELBOURNE AND NEW YORK 1983

CHURCHILL LIVINGSTONE
Medical Division of Longman Group Limited

Distributed in the United States of America by Churchill Livingstone Inc., 1560 Broadway, New York, N.Y. 10036, and by associated companies, branches and representatives throughout the world.

First Edition 1973
Second Edition 1983

ISBN 0 443 02610 6

British Library Cataloguing in Publication Data

Grenville-Mathers, R.
  The respiratory system. – 2nd ed. – (Penguin library of nursing series)
  1. Respiratory organs – Diseases
  2. Respiratory disease nursing
  I. Title
  616.2'0024613   RC731

Library of Congress Cataloguing in Publication Data

Grenville-Mathers, R. (Ronald)
  The respiratory system.
  (Penguin library of nursing)
  Bibliography: p.
  Includes index.
  1. Respiratory disease nursing. I. Title. II. Series
[DNLM: 1. Respiratory tract diseases – Nursing.   WY 163
G828r]
RC735.5.G73   1982   610.73'692   82-4121
                    AACR2

Printed in Singapore by Huntsmen Offset Printing Pte Ltd

The
Respiratory
System

Penguin Library of Nursing

Other books in the Series:

The Cardiovascular System
The Digestive System
The Endocrine System
The Female Reproductive System
The Neuromuscular System
The Musculoskeletal System
The Urological System
The Special Senses

The Penguin Library of Nursing Series was
created by Penguin Education and is
published by Churchill Livingstone

Preface

Respiration is vital to man's survival. Indeed, there are only two ways of dying – by the cessation of breathing or by cardiac arrest.

Diseases of the respiratory system are, therefore, very important and comprise about 25 per cent of medical practice today. In winter, outbreaks of respiratory disease fill the medical wards of our hospitals and even encroach on the surgical divisions.

Many of these diseases are preventable, but knowledge of the measures necessary is not widely disseminated. So, in the preparation of this book, we have endeavoured to present the causes, nursing care and treatment of the more common respiratory diseases for the benefit of nursing staff coming in contact with such cases.

The patient benefits if the attending staff appreciate the reasons why certain procedures are used, and this requires some knowledge of the underlying theory. I hope I have presented the necessary information in a simple, informative and interesting manner.

I particularly wish to thank my various Ward Sisters and a number of Tutors who have helped me through discussions of the problems encountered by nurses.

Invaluable help and a wealth of experienced advice has also been rendered to me by the publishers, to whom I am most grateful.

1983   R.G-M.

To ANWAR
My *Light of Lights*

Contents

1. The thorax   1

2. The symptoms of respiratory disease   21

3. Acute infections of the respiratory tract   30

4. Obstructive lung disease   45

5. Generalized diseases of the lung   74

6. Tumours of the chest   98

7. Diseases of the pleura and the diaphragm   129

Further reading   140

Index   142

One
The thorax

The respiratory system

Respiration is the act of breathing. We breathe in air through the nose and mouth, it then passes through the *pharynx* (the space at the back of the mouth), the *larynx* (or voicebox) situated at the front of the neck, through the *trachea* (or windpipe), and into the lungs. The upper part of the trunk which contains the lungs is called the *thorax* (Fig. 1.1).

The oxygen contained in the air we breathe is essential to life; without it we die in a matter of minutes. The cells of our bodies need oxygen to burn food in order to provide them with the energy

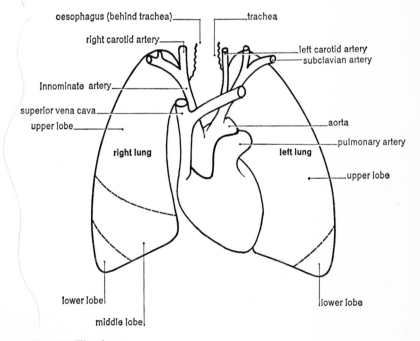

Fig. 1.1 The thorax

to carry out their functions. Another gas, carbon dioxide, is produced as a result of this process. It is poisonous in high concentra-
tions, and has to be removed from the body.

Man needs large amounts of oxygen to stay alive, and one of the
functions of the blood stream is to carry oxygen to the cells and to
bring back carbon dioxide (Fig. 1.2). The lungs provide the
mechanism by which these gases are exchanged. Each lung consists
of a large membrane folded many times in order to get a large surface area into a relatively small volume. The blood is on one side of
this membrane and the oxygen in the lungs is on the other. Because
the pressure of oxygen is lower in the blood than it is on the other
side of the membrane, oxygen passes through the membrane and
into the blood, where it dissolves. Carbon dioxide passes through
the membrane from the blood into the air in the lungs because the
pressure of the carbon dioxide is greater in the blood than in the
air.

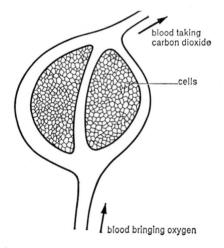

Fig. 1.2 The vascular system

The trachea and bronchi

The air reaches the lungs through a series of conducting tubes.
After the air has been filtered, warmed and saturated with water
vapour by the nose, it passes through the pharynx, the larynx and
down the trachea. This tube is kept rigidly open by rings of cartilage so that the air can always pass freely down it. These rings are
incomplete at the back where the *oesophagus* (gullet) lies against the
trachea. At its lower end, the trachea divides into two smaller

tubes, also ringed with cartilage, called the left and right main *bronchi*. The angle between the two main bronchi is called the *carina*. The right bronchus is shorter and more vertical than the left, so inhaled foreign bodies usually drop into this side. It divides into three branches, to the upper, middle and lower lobes of the right lung, while the left bronchus divides into only two, to the upper and lower lobes of the, slightly smaller, left lung. In these lobes, the tubes divide again and again, ending in tiny sacs called *alveoli*, where most of the gas exchange occurs. The whole arrangement is very much like a tree, the trachea forming the trunk and the bronchi forming the major boughs, which give off smaller and smaller branches (Fig. 1.3).

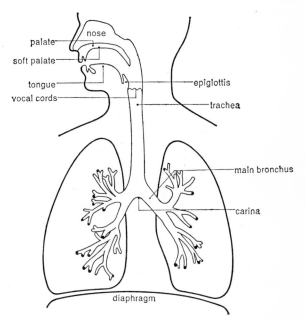

Fig. 1.3 The trachea and bronchi

Development of the lungs

The lungs did not originate in the thorax (the upper part of the trunk). In the foetus, a small ridge develops in the floor of the gut, and this is eventually cut off from the oesophagus, forming a separate tube leading into the pharynx just in front of the oesophagus. The upper part of this tube develops into the larynx and the trachea and the lower part into the lung bud, which then divides to form the left and right lungs (Fig. 1.4).

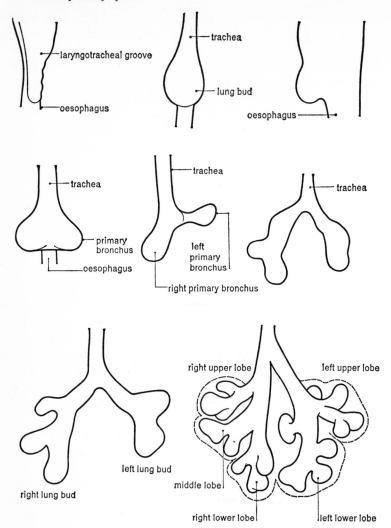

Fig. 1.4 Development of the trachea, bronchi and lungs

The tracheal tube gradually lengthens and becomes lined with a coating of cells called *columnar epithelium*. These cells (Fig. 1.5) have small hair-like projections (*cilia*) which trap any dirt particles reaching the trachea. The cilia are covered with *mucus*, which is produced by the bronchial glands and, as the cilia move (Fig. 1.6), the mucus sticks to the dirt particles, forming blebs which can be coughed up.

The lung buds give off bronchial buds soon after they are formed

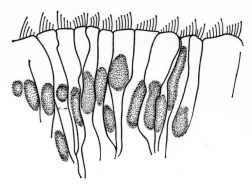

Fig. 1.5 Ciliated cells

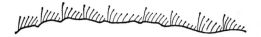

Fig. 1.6 Movement of cilia

and these will develop into the bronchial tree, the smallest branches terminating in the alveoli. The walls of these tiny sacs are pressed together during foetal life, and they only open up and start functioning at birth. When the baby is born, the bronchial buds have already divided eighteen times, and this branching process goes on until twenty-four divisions have occurred. This usually takes until middle childhood.

Until the baby is born, the lungs are relatively small, since they are not used. When the baby starts breathing, the lungs gradually expand to fill the lung cavity. (This is significant from the legal point of view, as it shows whether or not a newborn baby has breathed.) The lungs will have fully expanded by the fourth day of life, and then the lung margins will be rounded and the lung tissue will be light and spongy.

The thoracic cage

The *thoracic cage* protects the lungs, the heart and the great vessels. It is formed by the breast bone (*sternum*) anteriorly, by twelve thoracic vertebrae posteriorly, and by twelve ribs on each side. Above it are the muscles and structures in the root of the neck. Below it is the *diaphragm*, a sheet of muscle separating the thorax from the abdomen.

The sternum (Fig. 1.7) is made up of three parts, an upper sec-

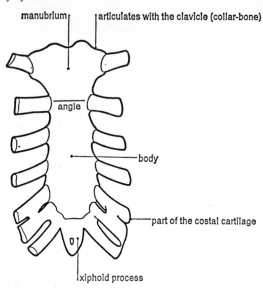

Fig. 1.7 The sternum

tion called the *manubrium*, a middle section called the *body* and a lower section called the *xiphoid process*.

Each of the twelve thoracic vertebrae or *dorsal vertebrae* (Fig. 1.8) has a small depression at the side for the head of the rib and a similar depression on the transverse process for the rib tubercle. The body of each vertebra is heart-shaped with a circular hole (the *vertebral foramen*) through which the spinal cord passes. The spine and the transverse processes on either side provide the attachments for the powerful back muscles.

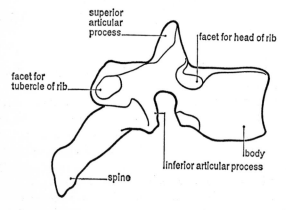

Fig. 1.8 Thoracic vertebra

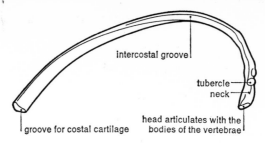

Fig. 1.9 A rib

The ribs themselves are curved, flat bones composed of a head, a neck, a tubercle and a shaft (Fig. 1.9). The upper seven pairs of ribs ('true ribs') are attached directly to the sternum by costal cartilages. The lower five pairs are called 'false' ribs. The first three pairs of these have their costal cartilages attached to those of the ribs above, and the remaining two pairs (the 'floating ribs') have no costal cartilages (Fig. 1.10). At the back, the head of the rib fits into the depression on the side of the thoracic vertebra, and the tubercle fits into the depression in the transverse process.

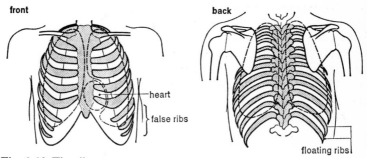

Fig. 1.10 The ribs

Occasionally an extra rib may develop in the neck, usually projecting from the seventh cervical vertebra. This *cervical rib* can cause pain and numbness in the arm because it may compress the nerves which supply the arm. These nerves arise in the neck and pass over the first rib, where the cervical rib can press on them.

Between each pair of ribs are the external and internal *intercostal muscles*. These, together with the diaphragm, are the muscles chiefly responsible for the movements involved in respiration. The external intercostal muscles arise from the lower border of a rib and pass to the upper border of the one below. The fibres of these mus-

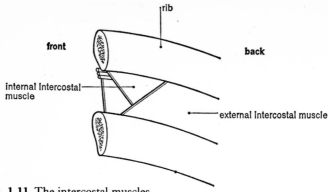

Fig. 1.11 The intercostal muscles

cles run obliquely forward (Fig. 1.11). The internal intercostal muscles lie inside the external intercostal muscles with their fibres running from front to back.

Along the lower border of each rib is a groove containing the intercostal artery, which supplies blood to the muscles in that rib space. The intercostal arteries are branches of the descending part of the thoracic aorta. Accompanying the artery are a vein and the intercostal nerve, which innervates the intercostal muscles. The blood vessels and nerve in this groove are thus protected from damage. Any needle inserted into the chest should go as close as possible to the bottom of the rib space to avoid damage to the blood vessels or to the nerve.

When the rib cage is relaxed, the head of the rib is higher than that of the top of the rib above. When the intercostal muscles contract they pull the ribs upwards and outwards (like the handle of a bucket), increasing the circumference of the thorax (Fig. 1.12).

The diaphragm

The diaphragm is a sheet of muscle separating the thorax from the abdomen. It is shaped like a dome and arises from the lumbar vertebrae, from the back of the lower part of the sternum and from the inner side of the lower six ribs. Its muscle fibres converge on a flat sheet of dense fibrous tissue known as the *central tendon* (Fig. 1.13). When these muscles contract, the central tendon is pulled downwards towards the abdomen. This lowers the pressure in the thorax and draws air into the lungs. When the muscles relax, the diaphragm rises again, pushing air out of the lungs (see Fig. 1.12).

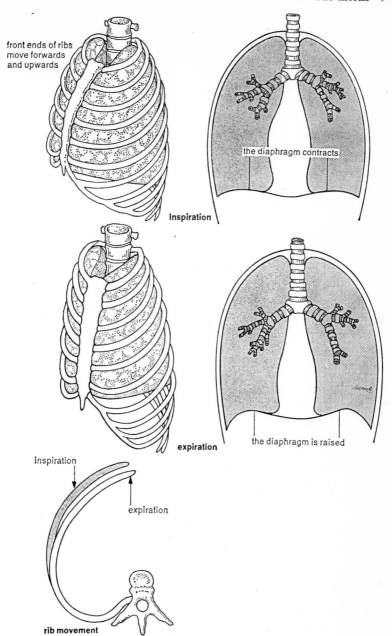

front ends of ribs
move forwards
and upwards

the diaphragm contracts

inspiration

the diaphragm is raised

expiration

inspiration

expiration

rib movement

Fig. 1.12 Respiration

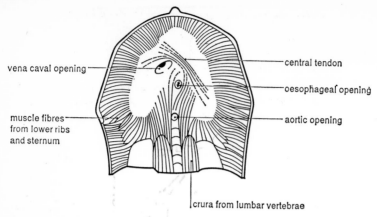

vena caval opening

muscle fibres
from lower ribs
and sternum

central tendon

oesophageal opening

aortic opening

crura from lumbar vertebrae

Fig. 1.13 The diaphragm

The nerve impulses which make the diaphragm contract flow through the *phrenic nerves* on either side of the diaphragm. These arise in the third, fourth and fifth cervical segments of the spinal cord and pass down the inner side of each lung to reach the diaphragm. Their action is controlled by the respiratory centre of the brain, which is in the medulla.

When breathing is difficult, the *accessory muscles* come into action (these normally move the head, arms and shoulder blades). When the arms and head are held steady, these muscles raise the front of the chest, increasing the volume inside. They consist of the *pectoralis major* muscle, which lies in the front wall of the chest, the *serratus anterior* muscle, which runs round the lateral wall of the chest, and the *sterno-mastoid* muscle, which passes from the back of the skull to the collar-bone. The abdominal muscles can also help breathing difficulty by pushing the diaphragm upwards when breathing out. In practice, most women use mainly the intercostal muscles (thoracic breathing) and men the diaphragm (abdominal breathing).

The lungs

The lungs, the organs of respiration, are situated on each side of the chest, separated by the heart, the aorta and the oesophagus. They are conical in shape, the apex rising into the root of the neck about two centimetres above the midpoint of the collar-bone (*clavicle*), the base resting on the diaphragm. The right lung is divided into three lobes, the upper, middle and lower lobes, and the left

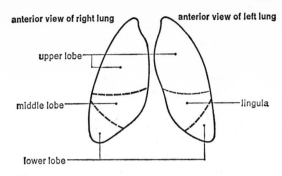

Fig. 1.14 The lungs

into two, the upper and lower lobes. The part of the left upper lobe that corresponds to the right middle lobe is known as the *lingula* (Fig. 1.14).

The root of the lung is on the medial surface and here the air tubes, the pulmonary artery and veins, the bronchial arteries and veins, and the pulmonary nerves all enter it. Each lobe is divided into a number of lobules consisting of a bronchial tube, air cells, blood vessels, lymphatics and nerves, all held together by connective tissue. The bronchial tubes end in a number of smaller tubes or bronchioles. Each of these terminates in an expansion called the *infundibulum*, off which branch the alveoli. These minute, pouch-like structures are arranged like a bunch of grapes, the bronchiole being the stem (Fig. 1.15). The many alveoli allow the large surface area of the lung to be stored in a compact space.

The very thin walls of the alveoli are made up of a single layer of cells (*pavement epithelium*). Each alveolus is surrounded by abundant blood capillaries (supplied with blood by the pulmonary arteries), so that there can be an easy exchange of oxygen and carbon dioxide. Oxygen is absorbed into the blood and taken up by the pigment *haemoglobin* in the red corpuscles. At the same time, the blood gives up the carbon dioxide which has been absorbed as waste matter from the cells. Water, too, passes out of the blood into the lungs, and is exhaled in the breath together with the carbon dioxide.

Each lung is surrounded by a continuous membrane, the *pleura*. The inner layer (the *visceral pleura*) closely covers the lung, passing into the fissures and separating the lobes. This membrane doubles back on itself at the root of the lung and forms the *parietal pleura* which covers the interior of the chest wall, the upper surface of the diaphragm, and the mediastinum. There is a space (the *pleural space*) between the two layers of pleura, and the pressure within

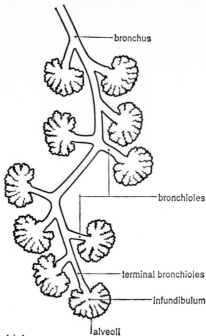

bronchus

bronchioles

terminal bronchioles

infundibulum

alveoli

Fig. 1.15 The bronchioles

this space is sub-atmospheric ('negative'). This is why, if a needle is inserted between the ribs and into the pleural spaces, air may be sucked in as the patient breathes.

How does the body get fresh air to the lungs? Air will only move from an area of high pressure to one of lower pressure. In breathing in (*inspiration*), the muscles cause the chest to expand, lowering the pressure of the air in the lungs below that in the nose and mouth. Consequently air is sucked in, down the trachea, bronchi and bronchioles to the alveoli. Breathing out (*expiration*) is a passive process, air being forced out of the lungs by their elastic recoil and by the muscles as they relax. In quiet breathing, the diaphragm contracts, thus enlarging the thorax downwards. When inspiration is a conscious effort, the intercostal muscles lift the ribs and sternum, expanding the thoracic cage at the sides, back and front. In severe exertion, when large amounts of oxygen are needed quickly, the accessory muscles of respiration expand the chest even further.

The control of breathing

Respiration is mainly an unconscious action controlled by nervous and chemical factors. If the spinal cord is cut low down in the neck,

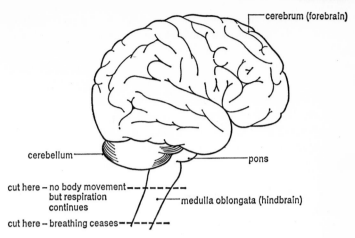

cerebrum (forebrain)

cerebellum

pons

cut here – no body movement
but respiration
continues

medulla oblongata (hindbrain)

cut here – breathing ceases

Fig. 1.16 The respiratory centre of the brain

all respiratory movements of the intercostal and abdominal muscles cease permanently. But, if the brain is cut across above the hindbrain (the *medulla oblongata*), respiration continues, indicating that there is a respiratory centre in the hindbrain (Fig. 1.16).

This respiratory centre automatically keeps breathing going at a steady rate. The rate may be altered by messages reaching the centre via the nerves and also by the chemical composition of the blood supplying the centre. Thus, breathing is quickened and deepened during bodily activity and slowed during sleep.

Nervous control

During inspiration, the walls of the bronchi become stretched. When a certain tension is reached, impulses pass from the bronchi via the *vagus* nerve (the tenth cranial nerve) to the respiratory centre. The centre then sends out nervous impulses to the intercostal and abdominal muscles, telling them to relax, and the natural elastic recoil of the lungs then expels air from the lungs – i.e. expiration occurs.

The endings of the vagus nerve in the bronchi may also be stimulated by irritating substances drawn into the air passages. This may cause wheezing, coughing or sneezing.

Chemical control

The respiratory centre is also affected by chemical agents in the blood supplying it, the most important of these being carbon dioxide. Any increase in carbon dioxide (such as results from increased muscular acitivity) stimulates the respiratory centre to greater activity so that breathing is quicker and deeper. (You can easily confirm this by breathing into a paper bag for a minute or so.)

In addition, the wall of the *carotid artery* (the main artery to the head) contains a structure called the *carotid sinus*. This is sensitive to an excess of carbon dioxide or a deficiency of oxygen in the blood, and nerve impulses from the sinus are sent to the respiratory centre to alter the rate and depth of breathing.

During rest, sixteen to eighteen breaths per minute are needed to supply the tissues of the body with sufficient oxygen and to get rid of excess carbon dioxide. The air in the alveoli normally contains around 5 to 6 per cent carbon dioxide. If a person voluntarily overbreathes, more carbon dioxide is removed from the body than usual. The respiratory centre loses one of its main stimuli to activity, and so respiration slows down until the right amount of carbon dioxide has again built up in the body. The nurse will quite often see patients who have overbreathed as a result of emotional stress, and have 'washed out' much of their carbon dioxide. These patients feel ill and very frightened and develop a peculiar spasm of the hands called 'tetany'. If the patient breathes into a paper bag, recovery will follow within a few minutes.

If a person breathes in more than about 10 per cent of carbon dioxide (as could happen if a child were to put its head into a plastic bag), dizziness occurs, followed by loss of consciousness. Similarly, if the oxygen content of the air breathed in is less than 13 per cent, the lack of oxygen is quickly felt. Breathing becomes more and more rapid, and eventually death will occur from asphyxiation.

Asphyxia is a condition in which the tissues are deprived of oxygen. As well as lack of oxygen, it can also result from the inability of the oxygen present to reach the different tissues of the body. Carbon monoxide (a gas produced by car engines) unites with the haemoglobin of the blood more readily than oxygen does, so if there is a high concentration of carbon monoxide in the air, as may occur if a car engine is run in a closed garage, the blood is unable to carry oxygen to the tissues, and asphyxiation and death result. Cyanide (prussic acid) also stops the haemoglobin of the blood giving up oxygen.

At the top of high mountains, the pressure of the atmosphere (and hence of the oxygen in it) is lower than at sea-level, consequently, adequate amounts of oxygen may not reach the blood. People not acclimatized to living at high altitudes will have to use the accessory muscles of respiration and increase their respiratory movements. After several months at high altitude, a person will develop an increased amount of haemoglobin in his blood, so that the blood can carry more oxygen.

The respiratory system must saturate the capillary blood with oxygen and excrete carbon dioxide in order to cope with activities ranging from resting in bed to running long distances. Therefore in assessing patients with respiratory disease, it is essential to know the precise efficiency of their respiratory function. There are three aspects to consider:

ventilation – the actual mechanism of getting air into and out of the alveoli;

gas exchange – the passage of oxygen and carbon dioxide through the alveolar membrane of the lung;

blood flow – the amount of blood passing through the lung capillaries.

Ventilation

In quiet respiration, the amount of air passing in and out of the lungs with each breath is known as the *tidal air* and can be measured using a *spirometer* (Fig. 1.17). When the patient breathes in and out of the mouthpiece, the cylinder moves up and down and the respiratory movements are traced on the revolving drum. Figure 1.18 shows the tracing obtained when the patient takes a deep breath in and then forces out of his lungs as much air as he can. The total amount of air which can be expelled in this way is called the *vital capacity*, and is a measure of the size of the lungs.

The average vital capacity for a young adult male is about 5 litres. It is usually lower in women, because they tend to be smaller, and it is higher in a trained athlete. The vital capacity also varies with body build and age, becoming less in old people.

Even after as much air as possible has been expelled from the lungs, some 1600 ml still remains in the alveoli. This is called the *residual air* and cannot be removed since the considerable pressure of the muscles on the chest wall causes the bronchioles in the lung to collapse, trapping the residual air.

The vital capacity is reduced in nearly all diseases of the lungs, pleura or thoracic cage. As a single test of respiratory function, measurement of the vital capacity has many limitations, mainly because it does not measure the *rate* at which a patient can expel air from his lungs. In an attempt to measure this rate, the forced vital capacity (FVC) is measured.

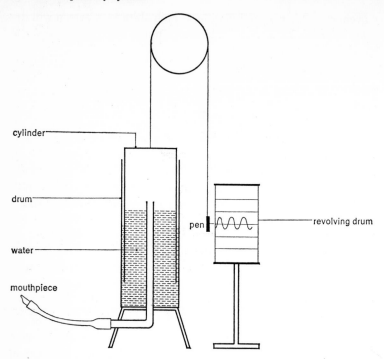

Fig. 1.17 A spirometer

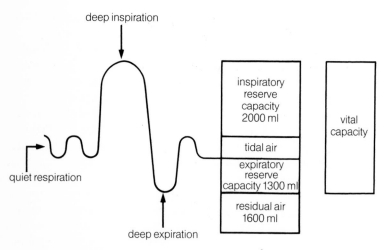

Fig. 1.18 A spirometer tracing

In this test, the patient inhales as deeply as possible, and then exhales as *rapidly* as he can. The total volume of air expelled (the FVC) and the amount of air expelled in the first second are measured on the spirometer. In a healthy person, at least 75 per cent of the FVC is expired in the first second. This is known as the forced expiratory volume in one second, and is usually written as FEV_1. The ratio FEV_1:FVC is an important measure of the degree of obstruction to ventilation in the bronchial tubes. This test is also valuable as a way of finding out whether anti-spasmodic drugs will help the patient. The measurement of the ratio FEV_1:FVC is so useful in estimating the ventilatory capacity of the lungs that single-breath machines have been produced which are used in place of a spirometer. Spirometers have many disadvantages, since they are not easily portable and are liable to spill water onto the ward floor. A most useful machine is the *vitalograph* (Fig. 1.19), which can be easily brought to the bedside. Its recording pen writes on special paper which is sensitive to pressure. The patient takes only one deep inspiration and breathes out as quickly as possible into the vitalograph tube. The paper is calibrated so that the FEV_1 and FVC can be read off immediately. Figure 1.20 shows an example of the tracing obtained.

Another test demonstrating the presence of obstruction to ventilation is the measurement of the *peak expiratory flow rate* (PEFR)

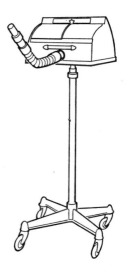

Fig. 1.19 A vitalograph

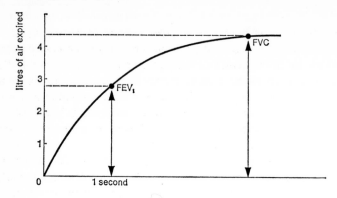

Fig. 1.20 A vitalograph tracing

using a Wright's Peak Flow Meter (Fig. 1.21). This measures the maximum rate of flow of air during a forced expiration. The result is expressed as the amount of air (in litres) which would be expired in one minute if the maximum rate of expiration could be maintained for that length of time. The apparatus is small, sturdy and easy to operate. A normal reading is between 400 and 600 litres per minute depending on the patient's sex, age and body size.

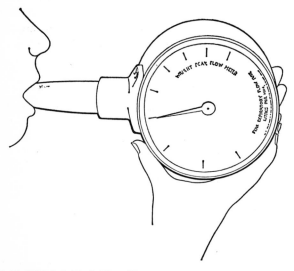

Fig. 1.21 Wright's Peak Flow Meter

Gas exchange

The tests described above are satisfactory ways of measuring the action of the lungs as a pair of bellows, but it is also necessary to find out if the air in the alveoli is being changed with each breath. This can be achieved by estimating the level of carbon dioxide in the alveolar air, using an electronic machine which automatically measures the percentage of carbon dioxide in the air breathed out. Alternatively, a sample of blood can be taken from an artery and its chemical content estimated.

In some diseases the air inspired is not evenly distributed through the lungs. This can be demonstrated by making the patient breathe from a bag of oxygen containing some radioactive xenon. A geiger counter is then placed over different parts of the lungs, and the number of clicks from the counter is a measure of the distribution of the gas in the lungs.

This method requires the services of a trained physicist, since radioactive material is being used. However, many hospitals use a nitrogen machine instead. The air we breathe is four-fifths nitrogen and one-fifth oxygen. If the inspired air is uniformly distributed through the lungs, the nitrogen will be also. In this test, the patient takes a deep breath from a bag containing pure oxygen, and then breathes out through a tube connected to a rapid nitrogen analyser. At first, the meter shows no nitrogen in the expired air (Fig. 1.22) since the air initially expelled comes from the trachea and the major bronchi, and is the pure oxygen which has just been breathed in. As expiration continues, the percentage of nitrogen steadily increases, becoming constant when 750 ml to 1250 ml of gas have been expired.

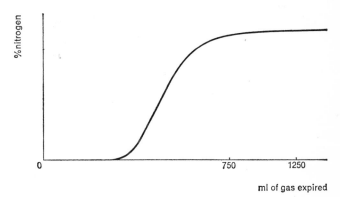

Fig. 1.22 Nitrogen wash-out technique

The efficiency of gas exchange through the alveolar membrane can be measured by determining the extent to which the haemoglobin in the blood has taken up oxygen. This can be measured directly by analysing blood withdrawn from an artery, but it is more easily performed using an instrument called an *oxymeter*. A clip is put on the lobe of the ear; on one side of the clip is a source of light, and on the other is a photo-electric cell which produces an electric current whenever a light shines on it. The size of the current provides an estimate of the amount of light passing through the ear lobe, and hence of the amount of oxygen being carried by the haemoglobin in the blood.

In some uncommon diseases, the failure of gases to pass through the alveolar membrane is of great diagnostic value. This failure can be demonstrated by measuring the rate of uptake of small amounts of carbon monoxide introduced into a bag of oxygen from which the patient breathes.

Blood flow

It may be necessary to determine the amount of blood passing through the lungs. A cardiac catheter is inserted into a vein in the elbow and passed along the vein, through the right atrium and right ventricle, until it reaches the pulmonary artery. Samples of blood are taken from the pulmonary artery and, at the same time, blood samples are taken from a peripheral artery. Simultaneously, the amount of oxygen breathed in by the patient each minute is measured. Since 100 ml of blood carries 20 ml of oxygen, the doctor can calculate the rate of flow of blood (in litres per minute) through the lungs.

Two
The symptoms of respiratory disease

The symptoms

There are only six symptoms of which the patient with a respiratory disease can complain. The way these symptoms develop and the order in which they occur give valuable clues to the diagnosis. It is important for the nurse to understand these symptoms, because the nursing team has the patient under observation throughout his stay in hospital while the medical staff are in the ward situation for brief periods only.

The six symptoms are:

1. Cough
2. Production of sputum
3. Coughing up blood (haemoptysis)
4. Shortness of breath (dyspnoea)
5. Pain in the chest
6. Loss of weight

1. Cough

This is a forced expiration against a closed throat. Air pressure in the trachea and bronchi is built up by fixing the chest muscles and tightening the diaphragm and the abdominal muscles. The throat is then suddenly opened and there is a rush of air from the peripheral parts of the lung towards the trachea. This pushes mucus towards the pharynx with an explosive discharge (producing the characteristic barking noise) and removes from the air passages any mucus or foreign particles which may have collected. Coughing is the main way in which the lungs are kept clean.

Like sneezing, coughing is a reflex action, but it can also be controlled voluntarily (children often cough to attract the attention of their parents). The cough reflex may be stimulated by irritation of the nerve endings in the larynx, trachea, bronchi and even the pleura, so a cough may not necessarily be due to disease in the lungs themselves. For example, a cough which is only present night and morning and on moving about is frequently due to the drip of nasal mucus into the pharynx. A cough is, however, a warning that disease may be present somewhere in the respiratory tract. This is particularly likely if the character of the cough has changed, becomes more frequent or produces more sputum. Although cigarette smoking is frequently associated with a cough, this may not be the main cause. It is not generally recognised that alcoholics have a cough, productive of sputum, that is most troublesome in the mornings. Nowadays, it is generally recognized that any patient who has had a cough for more than two or three weeks needs a chest X-ray. Persistent coughing is very wearing for the patient and those around him and the nurse may assist by encouraging a sitting up position, well supported by pillows: this allows maximum expansion of lung tissue. The diaphragm is able to contract freely without any restriction of movement from abdominal contents and as a result coughing is more effective. A dry rasping cough, non-productive of sputum may be relieved by an increase in the humidity of the atmosphere or warmth of the room or by administering cough suppressants or simply a hot drink. A deep cough productive of sputum needs encouragement. Expectorants may be prescribed. The aid of the physiotherapist will be enlisted to teach breathing exercises and institute postural drainage; alternatively a nebulizer may be used. The nurse needs to work as a team with the physiotherapy department and continue the treatment at night and at week-ends if the lungs are to be cleared of sputum. As nursing care is given throughout the day time, care must be taken to give the patient encouragement to cough and expectorate.

2. Production of sputum

The normal healthy adult does not produce sputum. Sputum is produced as a result of irritation of the respiratory tract (either by smoke, dust or bacteria). In the ward situation sputum is collected in a disposable plastic container with screw-on lid and the patient is instructed to keep the lid on when not in use. Every container in the ward should be collected at the same time each day, preferably after the consultants' round. A record should be made of the quantity, colour and any other characteristics, such as odour. The disposable containers are incinerated. A lot may be learned by observation of the sputum and it is a mistake to toss the container into the bag for incineration without first inspecting the contents. When planning the patients's care the nurse will take into account any aids to expectoration which may be deemed necessary, such as

steam inhalations or physiotherapy and the use of expectorants prescribed.

Specimens of sputum will be required for laboratory purposes
and it is important to get a good fresh specimen which has really
come from the respiratory passages and is not merely saliva. Early
morning is the best time to get a good specimen because the secretions have had time to collect overnight. In any event the aim is to
get a specimen which most accurately respresents the symptoms of
the patient concerned.

Patients with left-sided heart failure sometimes cough up large
amounts of clear, frothy sputum, which may be tinged with pink.
This is particularly liable to happen at night. While he is asleep, the
patient usually slips down in the bed, so the movement of the diaphragm is lessened and the heart cannot contract efficiently. The
vessels of the lung become engorged with blood, and fluid escapes
from the blood vessels into the alveoli producing acute shortness of
breath (*paroxysmal nocturnal dyspnoea*) and the characteristic sputum.

3. Coughing up blood (haemoptysis)

This is an important and common medical problem. The main difficulty is to distinguish it from the vomiting of blood (*haematemesis*), particularly as the account given by the patient may not always
be clear. The difference is usually obvious to the nurse observing
the patient at the time it occurs. Blood from the lungs is usually
bright red or pink, frothy and mixed with sputum. When the blood
comes from the stomach it is usually a darker colour and may be
mixed with food; if the blood has remained in the stomach for a little time, it resembles coffee grounds. In addition, the gastric fluid
is acid so that, if a nurse is in doubt as to whether haemoptysis or
haematemesis has occurred, blue litmus paper should be dipped
into the fluid. If the paper turns red, then the fluid is acid and
probably came from the stomach. Should there be any doubt, the
material must be saved for the doctor's inspection. The volume
must be measured, as it may be critical in a case of haematemesis.

Haemoptysis may be caused by over-violent coughing, pulmonary embolism, pneumonia, lung cancer, bronchiectasis, tuberculosis, mitral stenosis, left-sided heart failure or lung abscess. It is a
symptom which frequently alarms the patient, and much reassurance may be required. A chest X-ray is obligatory, and extensive
investigation may be needed in order to find the cause. In nearly
half the cases, however, no precise diagnosis can be made and the

investigations only serve to exclude the possibility of serious disease in the respiratory tract.

Where the haemoptysis consists only of the streaking of sputum it is sufficient for the nurse to report it to the medical staff at the earliest opportunity. Larger quantities of frank blood requires the patient to be put in the semi-recumbent position, call for medical aid, and whilst waiting record pulse and blood pressure and note the general condition. If the patient can tell from which side of the chest the bleeding is coming (and very often he can) he should be inclined gently to that side to prevent blood trickling into the sound lung.

4. Shortness of breath (dyspnoea)

This is a frequent symptom in respiratory disease, and is often difficult to evaluate since the doctor has only the patient's account to go on. The patient may say he is 'out of breath' or that he cannot fill his lungs, these symptoms constituting what is meant by shortness of breath. Unfortunately, there is no precise way of evaluating the patient's respiratory distress. Many patients with fairly good results in tests of respiratory function will complain bitterly of being short of breath, while others with worse results will hardly complain at all. Dyspnoea is obviously affected by emotion, ignorance, fatigue and other factors. People become more short of breath as they get older, and the only practical way of evaluating the symptom in the ambulant patient is by noticing whether he seems more breathless than other people of the same age when they are walking together. In the severely ill patient in bed, respiratory distress is usually obvious.

In pneumonia and *pleurisy* (inflammation of the pleura), breathing is rapid and shallow, and inspiration often stops abruptly (usually with an audible grunt) as soon as the pain ('pleuritic pain') is felt. A chronic bronchitic will often purse his lips while breathing out; in this way expiration is slowed and the bronchi are kept open longer so that more air can be expired. These patients are always more comfortable sitting up, either in bed or in an armchair: in either case they need to be well supported by pillows to enable them to relax, and they need to be encouraged to use the base of their lungs for breathing. Breathlessness over an extended period of time leads to immobility and stiffness of the joints which can increase the rehabilitation problems.

In patients with uraemia or uncontrolled diabetes, very deep, rapid breathing occurs, due to chemical stimulation of the respiratory centre of the brain. This condition is called 'air-hunger'. Cheyne–Stokes respiration is a characteristic rhythm which occurs when the respiratory centre loses its sensitivity to the concentration of carbon dioxide in the blood. The respirations become progressively deeper until a maximum is reached, and then diminish until there is an interval when no respiration occurs. The whole cycle lasts two or three minutes and is then repeated. This type of breathing occurs typically with failure of the left side of the heart (Fig. 2.1).

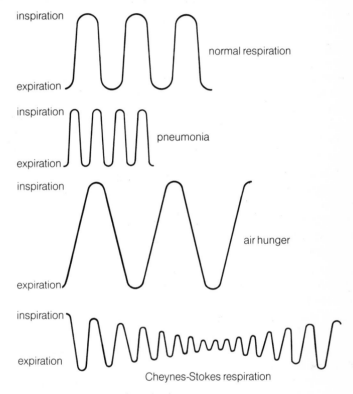

Fig. 2.1 Different types of respiration

5. *Pain in the chest*

The pain caused by pleurisy is sharp and stabbing and is made worse by deep breathing, coughing, sneezing and yawning, and particular movements such as turning the trunk and using the arms. The pain is usually localized at the site of the pleurisy, but it may be referred to the front of the abdomen, where it may be confused with an acute abdominal condition. When the pleurisy is located in the region of the diaphragm, the pain is often referred to the tip of the shoulder.

A rib fracture or the secondary deposit of a cancer in a rib can cause localized pain and tenderness and this, too, may be aggravated by breathing. Pain may also be experienced in the chest when a lesion is present in the spine.

Muscle or ligament strains often cause pain in the chest wall. These pains are not always recognised for what they are, and may be mistaken for symptoms of respiratory or cardiac disease.

Diseases of the heart, such as myocardial infarction and angina, can cause pain in the chest. So too can disease in the alimentary tract, such as hiatus hernia, a condition in which the stomach protrudes through the diaphragm into the chest. Some people with bronchial carcinoma complain of an ache in that part of the chest over the site of the neoplasm, but this is rare.

Emotional disorders commonly cause chest-wall pain, often described as a 'tightness'. It may be associated with palpitations, and alarm the patient considerably. The pain may occur below the left nipple (left sub-mammary pain) or over the sternum; confusion with heart disease may occur, but the association with fatigue or emotional strain is usually clear. The pain probably develops from unconscious tensing of the muscles. The nurse must be aware of the significance of (a) the time of onset; (b) the nature of the pain; and (c) the effect it has on the condition of the patient. Measuring pain takes experience and observation and there is only a very inexact and subjective opinion. The fact that a patient has asked for analgesics is an indication that all is not well; noticing his expression, the way he holds his hands and general demeanour, the condition of the skin, even the way he is breathing helps to evaluate pain. Patients frequently wait until they think it is convenient before they ask for analgesics: other factors may be 'waiting for their nurse' or their past experience. Are we always prompt in administering prescribed analgesics? Are we always sympathetic? One brusque reply from a nurse to a patient in such circumstances may prevent him from asking for relief in the future. Some patients having analgesics during terminal care can have their medications prescribed to be given at regular interval: in these circumstances the nurse should not ask if the patient is in pain, but simply give the drug following the routine safety procedure, because the philosophy of this type of treatment is to ensure that the patient never experiences pain and therefore eventually forgets what it feels like and therefore loses his fear of pain.

6. Loss of weight

This is not a common symptom at the beginning of acute infection but it is more marked in chronic illness of the respiratory tract. It is frequently an early symptom of pulmonary tuberculosis but only becomes noticeable in the late stages of a disease such as bronchial carcinoma. Wasting of the muscles (especially in the hands and arms) may be a particular feature of the latter condition.

Investigation of a patient with respiratory disease

The first stage in any investigation is for the doctor to take a careful history of the patient's symptoms. Patients are not always precise in the answers they give and frequently realize later that they have withheld useful information. The nurse, who is in close contact with the patient, will often obtain valuable information from him, frequently as a result of casual conversation. As a member of the diagnostic and therapeutic team, she should always report anything of significance that she learns in this way. Often it is the nurse who finds out that some member of the family has had tuberculosis, or that a workmate had developed this disease some time previously.

Clinical examination

After the doctor has taken the patient's history, he proceeds to the examination. The examination tray should contain a sphygmomanometer (for measuring blood pressure), cotton wool, pins, and ophthalmoscope, a patella hammer and a tuning fork in working order and a supply of disposable tongue depressors. The nurse should give assistance in cases where the patient is short of breath, distressed, unconscious or semiconscious and in the days of patient allocation and nursing process the nurse-patient relationship is enhanced by the sharing of this part of the admission procedure. The nurse should know what the patient recognises as his problems and what the doctor has said to the patient, and there is no better way of knowing this than being there at the examination: it also saves an ill and breathless patient having to repeat himself for the benefit of the nursing history sheet. A male doctor also needs a chaperone when examining a female patient.

The clinical examination is not confined to the chest, even if all the patient's symptoms are related to this area. For example, swelling and hardness in the leg may point to deep vein thrombosis as the cause for a pulmonary embolus. The doctor starts with a general inspection of the patient, dealing in turn with the hands, upper limbs, head, neck, chest, abdomen and the lower limbs. An important finding in diseases of the lungs and heart is *clubbing* of the fingers (see Fig. 5.10, p. 00). In this condition, the ends of the fingers are swollen and the skin becomes shiny, especially at the base of the nail, the nails themselves becoming much more curved. There are many causes of clubbing, including bronchial carcinoma, bronchiectasis, lung abscess, empyema, chronic pulmonary fibrosis and emphysema. It also occurs in diseases of the heart such as bacterial endocarditis and congenital heart disease, and in certain abdominal conditions.

General inspection of the chest may reveal abnormal curvature of the spine. *Kyphosis* (where the spine is bent forward) or *scoliosis* (where there is lateral bending) may alter the internal diameter of the chest (Fig. 2.2) and, in later years, give rise to severe impairment of lung function and even heart failure, but they are usually of no significance. Over-inflation of the lungs, which can occur in emphysema and asthma, makes the chest barrel-shaped.

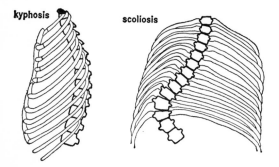

Fig. 2.2 Deformities of the chest

The doctor will note the respiratory rate, since this is increased in acute and chronic lung disease, heart failure and anxiety. It is decreased where the respiratory centre in the brain is depressed by poisoning or by various diseases of the brain. If there is severe respiratory disease, as in an asthmatic attack, the accessory muscles of respiration are used, including the pectoralis major and the sternomastoid.

The doctor also *palpates* the chest with his hands and assesses the degree of expansion at each breath. He then *percusses* the chest, laying one finger of his left hand flat on the skin and hitting the finger with the middle finger of his right hand. The sound produced in this way gives a valuable indication of the condition of the underlying lung.

He will now use a stethoscope on the chest to listen for the breath sounds as the air goes into and out of the lung. These sounds are altered in various diseases, and sometimes additional noises can be heard. For example, if pleurisy is present, a pleural rub can usually be elicited and, if bronchitis is present, scraping, rattling or wheezing noises may be heard.

In all cases of respiratory disease, chest X-rays are required. In addition, the movements of the chest and diaphragm can be observed under the X-ray screen. Other tests will depend on the disease suspected, and will be dealt with in the following chapters.

Three
Acute infections of the respiratory tract

About 20 per cent of all illnesses seen by doctors in Great Britain are respiratory diseases. Atmospheric pollution is a major cause of many of these. For instance, the great London 'smog' of 1952 caused 4000 deaths from respiratory disorders in four days, and many patients living in London still relate their respiratory troubles to that time. In the last twenty years, Governments in many countries have taken anti-pollution measures designed to control the emission of smoke from both industrial and domestic fuel-burning apparatus.

Other factors which may increase the incidence of respiratory disease include high atmospheric humidity, cold weather and the presence of pollen in the air. Cigarette smoke is also of immense importance in producing respiratory disease.

Dust, pollen and bacteria are trapped in the nose when a person breathes in. The nose does not remove all the irritants, however, and people who breathe through the mouth have no protection at all. The inhaled particles are normally trapped by the ciliated epithelium of the bronchi and eventually coughed up. In the healthy person this is a very efficient mechanism, and usually no bacteria can be cultivated from the secretions in the trachea and major bronchi. But this is not so where these primary defences fail to prevent organisms passing down the trachea and bronchi.

Acute tracheobronchitis

This is common in cool, damp climates. Men are affected more frequently than women because they tend to smoke more tobacco and are more often exposed to irritants in the atmosphere at work. The condition is more common in infancy and old age, and attacks occur mainly in winter, late autumn and early spring. The initial infection is usually by a virus, although secondary bacterial invasion of the trachea and the bronchi usually occurs.

An attack often begins suddenly with a feeling of being unwell, aching in the limbs and a heavy feeling in the chest. If the trachea is chiefly involved, there is a feeling of rawness behind the breastbone. The temperature rises to 37.8° C (100.0° F) in mild cases, or 39.4° C (102.9° F) in more severe cases. A dry, irritating cough develops, and this becomes looser in a few hours.

At first the sputum is scanty, sticky and white or grey in colour, but it becomes profuse, frothy and mucoid. Occasionally it is streaked with blood. As soon as the sputum becomes profuse, the symptoms diminish: the feeling of rawness behind the breastbone disappears and the soreness round the chest and lower ribs subsides. The temperature usually settles within five to six days (Fig. 3.1), but the cough and sputum may continue for ten days or more, gradually diminishing (with the sputum becoming thick and yellow) until they are present only at night and in the morning, finally disappearing altogether. In flu epidemics, the cough and sputum may last for some weeks before clearing up completely. In some patients the inflammation, instead of clearing up, spreads further down the respiratory tract to affect the finer bronchi and

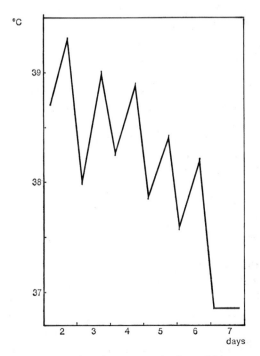

Fig. 3.1 Temperature chart in acute tracheobronchitis

bronchioles. Repeated attacks may result in the development of chronic bronchitis.

Treatment

Prophylatic. When giving general advice on health to patients with chest trouble, nurses should stress that crowded places of entertainment and ill-ventilated rooms should be avoided when catarrhal infections are at their peak during the winter time. Children should be encouraged to play in the open air and should be dressed in warm clothes, but not over-clothed. Damp clothes should be changed as quickly as possible. Mouth-breathers should be encouraged to take periodic deep breaths through the nose and to seek further medical attention for the nose and throat.

In dusty occupations, measures can be taken to reduce the amount of irritants in the atmosphere by employing extractor fans, and the factory nurse should encourage the use of gas masks where necessary. All patients, and particularly those who have chest disease, should be discouraged from smoking.

Curative. All patients with acute bronchitis should remain in bed until their temperature has returned to normal, and they should stay in a warm atmosphere for some days afterwards. They should have plenty of hot drinks and inhalations of medicated steam –5 ml of Tinct.Benz.Co. or 10 ml of pine oil to 500 ml of water at 70° C – help to relieve the soreness behind the sternum.

An antibiotic is usually given as soon as possible. Amoxycillin (250 mg four times a day) is often considered the best, since the most common organisms involved in secondary bacterial infection, the *pneumococcus* and *Haemophilus influenzae*, are both sensitive to the drug.

If the cough is very irritating at the start of the illness, it may be soothed by sipping 5 ml of syrup codeine phosphate mixed with an equal quantity of hot water. A sedative may also be necessary at night. There is no need for expectorants to be given. As the cough becomes more productive, encouragement should be given and the position changed frequently to enable secretions from all areas of the bronchial tree to drain into a situation from which they may be expectorated easily. The elderly experience more difficulty in summoning the muscular strength to cough effectively under these conditions and retained secretions will prolong the illness and predispose to bronchopneumonia.

A gradual return to former activities is prudent – the elderly requiring a longer period of convalescence.

The pneumonias

Pneumonia is a general term applied to any inflammation of the lung substance, whatever the cause. The pneumonias can be divided into two groups:

a. Those which are caused by a specific organism (such as the pneumococcus, the streptococcus or a virus) and result in diffuse infection of a lobe or lobes (Fig. 3.2); the term *lobar pneumonia* is applied to this type.

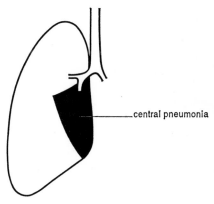

central pneumonia

Fig. 3.2 Lobar pneumonia

b. Those in which some abnormality of the lungs or respiratory tract predisposes them to invasion by organisms from the nose and throat. There is usually a gradual spread down the trachea, resulting in patchy areas of inflammation in both lungs. This type is often referred to as *bronchopneumonia* (Fig. 3.3).

Lobar pneumonia

This disease (also known as pneumococcal pneumonia) is characterized by the consolidation of one or more large segments or lobes of the lung. The pleura over the affected area is usually inflamed. The affected lobe consolidates and exudes fibrin and red and white blood cells into the alveoli. The disease clears up when the exudate liquefies and is either absorbed or expectorated. As the infected sputum is coughed up, droplets may be inhaled by other people, so the disease spreads. The incubation period is between two days and a week.

The onset of the disease is acute and sudden – so sudden that the patient can often recall the precise hour at which the illness began. He feels feverish and unwell, and may shiver uncontrollably. A

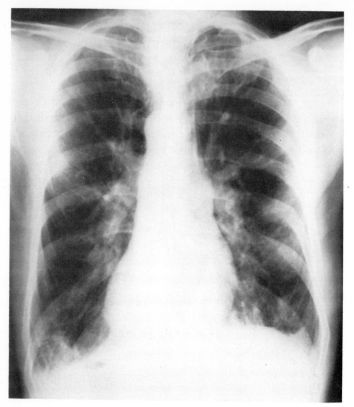

Fig. 3.3 The lungs in bronchopneumonia

short, dry, irritating cough develops, accompanied by a severe stabbing pain in the side. Breathing becomes rapid and shallow. At first the sputum is scanty and very sticky, but in a day or two it becomes more abundant and characteristically rusty in colour. In some patients, the sputum is thinner and looks like prune juice.

Herpes simplex (cold sores) may appear around the mouth. The temperature rises abruptly reaching 39.4° C (102.9° F) or even 40.5° C (104.8° F), as shown in Figure 3.4. A blood count shows a rise in the polymorphonuclear white cells (white cells with segmented nuclei), and a chest X-ray shows a diffuse haziness over the affected lobe. The pneumococcus can be isolated from the sputum.

In children there is rarely any obvious sputum, since it is swallowed. Vomiting and convulsions are common at the beginning of the illness. Infection of the ear is a frequent complication.

In old people, the onset is usually slow and the disease may be

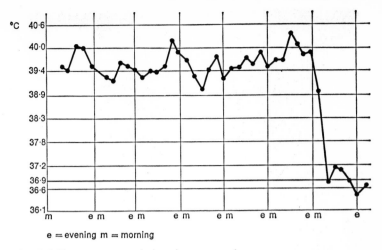

e = evening   m = morning

Fig. 3.4 Temperature variations in pneumonia

advanced before the diagnosis is made. Pneumococcal pneumonia is
a serious disease, especially in alcoholics and those with diabetes
mellitus, chronic heart disease, marked debility, or obesity.

Post-operative and traumatic pneumonia. Lobar pneumonia commonly occurs after surgical operations. In these cases, the condition
arises partly because pain limits the movement of the chest and
partly because collapse of a lobe may occur as a result of depression
of the cough reflex, general weakness and the inhalation of pus or
vomit.

Traumatic pneumonia frequently follows a chest injury. Some
cases are due solely to haemorrhage into the lung substance, but in
others bacterial infection is superimposed – the disease may then be
very serious.

Staphyloccal pneumonia. This is due to infection with *Staphylococcus
pyogenes*. It is usually a complication of other staphylococcal infections such as boils or abscesses, but in some cases the site of this
primary infection cannot be determined (Fig. 3.5). Patchy consolidation of the lung occurs, with a tendency to form thin-walled
cavities which look like soap bubbles on the X-ray.

The disease starts insidiously, and progresses rapidly with high
fever and sweating. If an abscess bursts into a bronchus, pure pus
is coughed up. Rupture into the pleura leads to the development of
an empyema or pyopneumothorax (see p. 131).

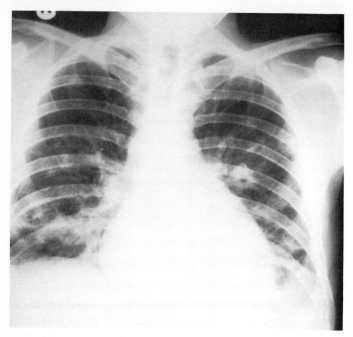

Fig. 3.5 Staphylococcal pneumonia

Friedlander's pneumonia. Friedlander bacilli are found among the normal flora of the mouth and intestinal tract and cause 1 per cent of all bacterial pneumonias. This disease is most common in men over the age of forty, especially in alcoholics.

The disease has similar features to pneumococcal pneumonia, with a sudden onset of chills, fever and pleuritic pain. The patient seems more severely ill, and the sputum is plentiful and *purulent* (contains pus). *Cyanosis* (a blue complexion due to lack of oxygen in the blood) and dyspnoea develop rapidly, and jaundice is often present. The upper lobe of the lung is frequently affected and cavity formation is common.

The fatality rate is high. A combination of antibiotics is usually necessary in treatment, and these are continued for at least ten to fourteen days.

Legionnaires' disease. This is a type of pneumonia which first became recognised in 1976, after a conference of the Americal Legion in Philadelphia. A large number of cases occurred with many deaths. The cause was not known until a new bacterium *Legionella pneumophilia* was identified. This does not give positive cultures with conventional methods but culture is now possible with the development of suitable media and a serological test is available.

The organism is carried in water but inhaled in showers and from air cooling systems. There have been outbreaks among groups such as holiday makers and sporting groups but sporadic cases do occur.

The disease starts with a mild respiratory infection which suddenly worsens with high fever, confusion, cough and diarrhoea. The disease is frequently rapidly progressive with a fatal ending, sometimes within 24 hours.

The treatment of choice is erythromycin, 500 mg every six hours, but is frequently ineffectual.

Treatment of lobar pneumonia

The patient is nursed sitting up in bed in a well-ventilated side room in which the temperature is maintained at 15.5–18.5° C (60 to 66° F). He should be disturbed as little as possible and given only fluids (2½ to 3 litres in 24 hours) in the acute stage. Milk or dextrose orangeade (dextrose 100 g, the juice of an orange and water to 500 ml) are suitable. This increased fluid intake compensates for fluid lost through perspiration and facilitates the expectoration of sputum. After a day or two, bread and butter, a boiled egg, or steamed fish can be given. Elderly patients may become incontinent, so, as a last resort a catheter should be inserted in the bladder and connected to a drainage bottle. A pad or towel should be placed under the buttocks if there is incontinence of faeces.

Debilitated patients may be too weak to cough up their sputum, and a physiotherapist can help here by positioning the patient in such a way that the diseased part of the lung is uppermost. If she places her left hand on this part of the chest and bangs the hand with the clenched fist of her other hand, the sputum will be expelled from the lung. In extreme cases, a catheter is inserted into the nose and pushed down into the trachea (Fig. 3.6). A syringe is then attached to the upper end of the tube and the sputum sucked out. The aspirating tube can then be pushed down into the left and right main bronchi by making the patient lean over to the appropriate side.

If the patient is cyanosed, he may be given oxygen (Fig. 3.7) by means of a catheter inserted into the nose or through a plastic face mask (*polymask*). The oxygen should be bubbled through a bottle of water before reaching the patient so that it contains a good deal of moisture to prevent drying of the respiratory tract.

The irritating cough can be checked if the patient sips a mixture

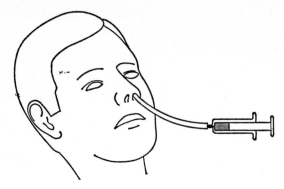

Fig. 3.6 A nasal catheter

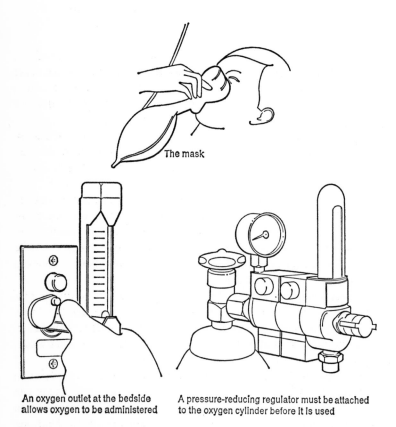

The mask

An oxygen outlet at the bedside allows oxygen to be administered

A pressure-reducing regulator must be attached to the oxygen cylinder before it is used

Fig. 3.7 The administration of oxygen

of 10 ml of syrup codeine phosphate in an equal quantity of hot water. Pleuritic pain may be relieved by injections of morphine (15 mg) or pethidine (50 mg) intramuscularly every six hours, and the application of local heat to the affected area of the chest. Observation of temperature, pulse, respiration and blood pressure are recorded four-hourly. A fall in temperature accompanied or not by a fall in blood pressure and pulse may indicate further spread of infection. Respiratory excursion is noted; this will be limited by the degree of infection and or the pleuritic pain. The characteristics of the sputum are recorded to give an indication of the progress of the disease and the response to antibiotics.

Physical rest is ensured to reduce the patient's oxygen demands. Time should be given between nursing treatments for undisturbed periods. An adequate explanation must be provided by the physician and elaborated upon by the nurse to allay anxiety.

Fever may be reduced by tepid sponging – the perspiration necessitates frequent change of clothing and bed linen.

Frequent small drinks help to keep the mouth fresh and clean, but more formal treatment may be indicated. The herpes that form during the later stages of the disease cause much tiredness and discomfort. Characteristically they resist all forms of treatment and run their course whatever is applied to them.

The patient must be encouraged to move his legs in the bed to prevent possible venous thrombosis. If he is too weak to do this, the nurse must bend and straighten his hip, knee and ankle joints several times every two hours.

Antibiotics are always given and have helped enormously in the treatment of this disease. An antibiotic given on the first day of illness will often bring the temperature down to normal within 24 to 48 hours and will also reduce the pulse and respiration rates. The general condition of the patient rapidly improves, pain is relieved and the toxic symptoms disappear.

A specimen of sputum is usually sent to the laboratory for culture to discover the responsible organism and to investigate its sensitivity to antibiotics. Meanwhile, treatment is started with intramuscular injections of benzyl penicillin (1 million units twice daily) or with amoxycillin (250 mg four times a day) by mouth.

If the patient is slow to recover, there may be some underlying disease such as bronchiectasis or carcinoma. A pleural effusion can occur as a complication of pneumonia; this is treated by aspiration and the injection of an antibiotic such as penicillin. If the fever recurs in spite of antibiotic treatment, the fluid in the pleural cavity may have become infected.

As soon as the temperature has subsided, the patient is encouraged to breathe as deeply and frequently as possible in order to promote full expansion of the lungs.

Virus pneumonias

These are not very common, except in epidemics. The incubation period for *atypical pneumonia* is usually from seven to fourteen days, and the onset is usually insidious, with a slight dry cough, mild chest discomfort, malaise and a moderately raised temperature. Physical examination of the chest generally reveals no abnormalities, but an X-ray often shows extensive mottled patches in both lungs (Fig. 3.8). A specific diagnosis can only be made by sending sputum for virus cultures, but the patient may have been discharged before the results are available.

Mild cases frequently recover spontaneously with symptomatic treatment such as linctus for the cough and inhalations of Friar's balsam. In more severe cases, an antibiotic such as amoxycillin is often given although it is doubtful if this drug does any good, since viruses are not susceptible to antibiotics.

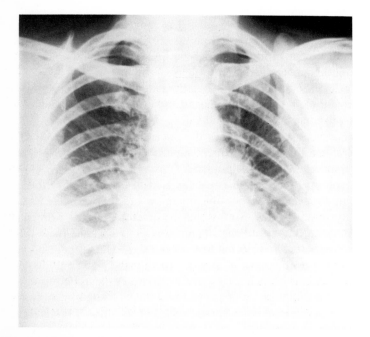

Fig. 3.8 The lungs in virus pneumonia

An uncommon pneumonia is *primary influenzal pneumonia*, which is a severe and usually fatal disease. Within 24 hours of the onset of the symptoms of influenza, the temperature rises to around 41° C (107° F). Cyanosis is marked and there is extreme dyspnoea and prostration. The cyanosis becomes deeper and takes on a heliotrope colour. The patient usually dies within five to ten days. Fortunately, this alarming clinical picture has not been seen on a widespread scale since the influenza pandemic of 1918–19. Nowadays the disease seems to be restricted mainly to patients with mitral stenosis.

Psittacosis is another rare virus illness. The psittacosis agent is a minute parasite which lives inside living cells. It is not really a true virus, being larger than most ordinary viruses (which is why it is susceptible to antibiotics). Parrots, budgerigars and canaries are commonly infected, but the agent is also found in turkeys, pigeons, ducks and chickens. People working with birds are most likely to become infected, and there is an increased incidence in pet shop employees and poultry workers.

Psittacosis causes a severe form of pneumonia with patchy consolidation of both lungs and, often, enlargement of the spleen. The condition usually responds well to tetracycline.

Acute bronchopneumonia

In bronchopneumonia, consolidation occurs in patches around the infected bronchi. It is usually found in the very young or the elderly and debilitated, and is due to the invasion of the lung by a mixture of the organisms normally present in the throat. In children, it often complicates measles and whooping cough.

The bronchi become acutely inflamed, and the terminal bronchioles are full of pus. Collapse of some alveoli and consolidation of others follows. Sometimes a large bronchus is blocked and *atalectasis* (collapse) of a segment or whole lobe occurs. The mortality is higher in the very young and very old.

The patient first shows the signs and symptoms of acute bronchitis but, as pneumonia develops, the temperature rises, the pulse and respiration rate increase and there is dyspnoea and cyanosis. There is a severe cough with purulent sputum, the culture of which produces only upper-respiratory-tract flora. The disease tends to run a longer course than lobar pneumonia, although the onset is less dramatic and the recovery is slower. Incomplete recovery may lead to bronchiectasis.

Treatment usually involves giving a wide-spectrum antibiotic such as tetracycline, ampicillin or septrin until the results of sputum culture and sensitivity tests are available. Postural drainage and physiotherapy should be instituted early in the disease.

Control of infection

Bacterial and viral pneumonias are communicable diseases; they are transmitted to others through droplet infection. Debilitated people will succumb more readily than those in good health.

The normal rules of hygiene are required, that the patient covers his mouth when coughing, uses paper handkerchiefs which can be burnt after use and all sputum is disposed of in a safe and acceptable fashion.

The nurse protects her uniform with a gown and wears a mask whilst attending to the patient and is careful to wash her hands after completion of her task. Visitors are kept to a minimum, firstly because the patient tires quickly, secondly to avoid unnecessary risk of spreading infection.

In severe cases, fever toxicity and hypoxia may give rise to confusion requiring the attendance of a nurse at all times and the use of cot sides on the bed. Sedation may be necessary to limit overexertion and further increase the O_2 demands. A drug such as valium which does not suppress the respiratory centre or the cough reflex will be prescribed.

As the temperature subsides activity is increased. The period of time taken for convalescence will vary depending on:
 (i) Severity of the illness
 (ii) The age of the patient
(iii) Complications, if any
In any event the patient will find he tires very easily, needing more rest than usual. He should avoid contact with anyone suffering from respiratory tract infections because his resistance to infection will be low.

In the absence of obesity a high protein diet may be recommended. The date of his return to work will be determined by his occupation.

Complications

These are rare in patients who are treated promptly and are not disadvantaged by underlying disease.

Atelectasis. This term describes collapse of a lobe or segment distal to a plug of mucus or similar obstructing a bronchial tube. Breathlessness and cyanosis develop causing restlessness. Examination of the chest shows little movement on the affected side and the radiograph demonstrates increased opacity. Atelectasis caused by retaining secretions can be avoided with adequate physiotherapy, deep breathing and assistance with coughing. Steam inhalations help to liquefy sputum and make it easier to expectorate.

Septicaemia. The causative organism may spread via the bloodstream giving rise to endocarditis, pericarditis, meningitis or arthritis. Blood Cultures will be taken and the chemotherapy altered to take care of this new development.

Empyema. See page 70.

Other infections

Aspergillosis A fungus which can infect the lungs is *aspergillus*. It is widely distributed but, fortunately, is an infrequent cause of disease. Two distinct conditions may be produced – asthma and mycetoma.

Asthma is dealt with in Chapter 4.

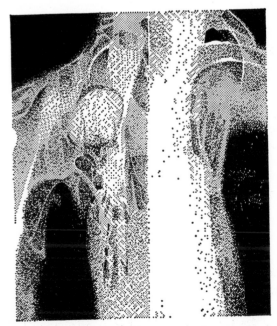
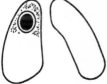

Fig. 3.9 An X-ray showing mycetoma in aspergillosis

Mycetoma is a swelling formed from a solid ball of fungus (Figure 3.9). This swelling is only found in lungs which have already been damaged by some other disease, such as tuberculosis or bronchiectasis. Treatment usually involves the removal of the damaged area of lung, but it may be best to leave the mycetoma untreated, merely taking routine X-rays from time to time.

Moniliasis. This is caused by *Candida albicans*, a yeast which frequently infects the mouth or the vagina. Administration of antibiotics to a patient may encourage its spread to other parts of the body – particularly the trachea and bronchi. Opinions differ on whether actual lung infection can occur, but monilial infection can certainly produce cough and dyspnoea. Treatment is by inhalations of nystatin, or Fluocytosine (Alcoban) 200 mg per Kg body weight daily, in four divided doses.

Mycoplasma. More cases of pneumonia are now occuring due to infection with mycoplasma. The distress can vary considerably in severity. The X-ray shows patchy shadows and the diagnosis is confirmed by a serological test. The disease responds to tetracycline 200 mgs or Erythromycin 500 mgs four times a day for six days.

Four
Obstructive lung disease

There are two main diseases which result from generalized obstruction in the bronchial tree, chronic bronchitis with emphysema, and asthma. In both diseases the patient has difficulty in expiring air, although the exact position of the obstruction in the bronchi is not known. It probably occurs throughout the smaller bronchi, which are not held open by the presence of rings of cartilage in their walls. This obstruction is aggravated by the presence of excess mucus in the bronchi.

In *choronic bronchitis*, respiratory function tests show that the obstruction is present all the time, whereas in *asthma* the obstruction is only present during an attack; between attacks, the lungs are perfectly normal.

Chronic bronchitis

A patient with advanced chronic bronchitis is a sorry sight. His face is pinched, his lips are blue, he has a distressing cough and is very short of breath, even when sitting in a chair. Dressing in the mornings may take over two hours. When he was younger, he probably had only a slight morning cough, which he may have attributed to smoking. The symptoms gradually progress over the years until they begin to interfere seriously with his normal life. The journey to work becomes increasingly difficult. Stairs are difficult to manage. Running for a bus becomes impossible and eventually he has to get up earlier because of the time taken to dress.

It is difficult to say at what point this condition should be labelled as chronic bronchitis. In general, the term is applied to patients who have morning cough and sputum every winter, provided that other causes (such as tuberculosis or bronchiectasis) have been excluded.

The disease is important because of the great disability it causes the sufferer and because of the economic consequences to the community. It is relatively uncommon in rural areas. In Europe, it is comparatively rare in Scandinavia, and even rarer in France and Switzerland. It is fairly common in the more industrial countries such as West Germany, Holland and Belgium and very common in the British Isles (Fig. 4.1), where it occurs in a belt running from the London area through the Midlands to the industrial North West. Its high frequency in the United Kingdom is associated with gross air pollution and a high incidence of cigarette smoking. Infections by viruses and bacteria may be important causes, but no definite relationship has been established. The disease is more common in men, particularly the middle aged and elderly.

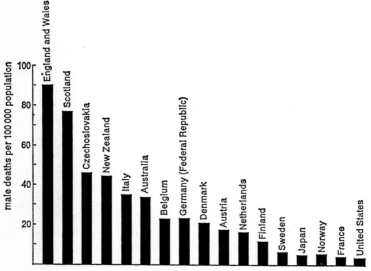

Fig. 4.1 Mortality from bronchitis. Figures (for 1964) supplied by the World Health Organisation

Most cases of chronic bronchitis could be prevented if atomospheric pollution could be reduced to nil, and if everyone gave up smoking.

In chronic bronchitis, the mucous membrane of the bronchi becomes inflamed and interferes with the smooth action of the cilia. This destroys the mechanism by which the lower respiratory tract is kept sterile. The epithelium of the bronchi becomes flattened (Fig. 4.2) and the number of cells bearing cilia is reduced. The mucus secreting glands in the bronchi increase and enlarge, which

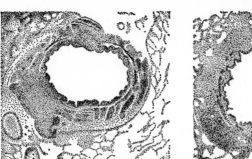
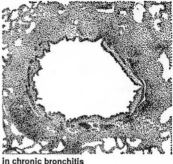

normal   in chronic bronchitis

Fig. 4.2 Transverse section of a bronchus

is why such a large amount of mucus is expectorated each day by chronic bronchitics. Eventually, some of the bronchioles become blocked with mucus, causing that portion of the lung they supply to collapse.

The obstruction traps air in the alveoli. These distend and many of them rupture, forming large irregular cysts (*bullae*) in the lung. This means that the amount of alveolar membrane available for gas transfer between the blood and the air in the lungs is diminished. The capillary bed of the lungs is also seriously reduced. Infection leads to widespread destruction of the bronchioles. The lungs lose their elasticity and increase in volume becoming *emphysematous* (inflated). This term is used when there is enlargement of the terminal air spaces of the lung, accompanied by destructive changes. Later the strain of respiratory impairment, the lack of oxygen and particularly the reduction in the number of capillary channels of the pulmonary vasculature causes hypertrophy and strain on the right side of the heart. This eventually leads to the development of congestive cardiac failure.

The characteristic sputum of a chronic bronchitic is a thick, tenacious mucus. This is often copious, and at times may be purulent. The microorganisms found in it vary, but *Haemophilus influenzae* and pneumococci are the most common secondary invaders of the rich mucus secreted by the hypertrophied glands.

Diagnosis

In the early stages of chronic bronchitis, an X-ray of the chest does not show any change. Only the larger bronchial tubes cast a shadow on a film, and the streaky pattern usually seen is due to the blood vessels. Sometimes this pattern is more prominent than usual, indicating dilated pulmonary vessels. In the later stages the ribs are seen to be widely spread and the heart shadow appears small. Bullae, or large air spaces, can often be seen and, if these become large and numerous, little normal lung pattern can be seen on the film (Fig. 4.3) – the vanishing lung syndrome. The main value of a chest X-ray in a patient complaining of chronic cough, sputum and wheezing is not to diagnose chronic bronchitis, but to exclude other causes of the symptoms, e.g. lung cancer.

A chronic bronchitic is usually slow in his movements. He may be cyanosed and appear slow-witted in answering questions. His chest may be barrel-shaped, but this is not always so. Chest expansion is usually poor. A characteristic finding is 'pursing' of the lips. These patients find difficulty in emptying their lungs in order to take in another breath. If expiration is rapid, the air pressure in the bronchial tubes falls rapidly, and so these tubes tend to collapse, trapping air in the alveoli. The bronchitic patient, by keeping his lips close together, lets the air out of his lungs slowly and so man-

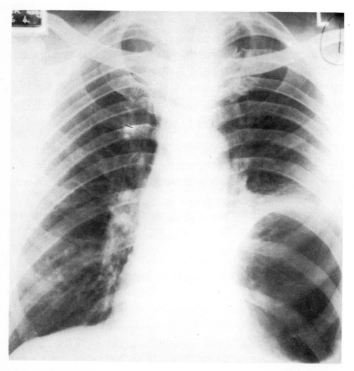

Fig. 4.3 An X-ray showing a large emphysematous bulla at the base of the left lung, with compression of the area of the lung above it.

ages to expire more air than if he allowed the air to escape quickly. This disease is therefore often referred to as one of chronic obstructive airway disease.

The disease is diagnosed mainly on the symptoms, on the fact that the chest X-ray does not reveal the presence of any other disease, and on the respiratory function tests. These tests are invaluable in diagnosing expiratory airway obstruction and assessing its progress. The obstruction in the bronchi, as explained above, is caused by weakening of their walls (which causes them to collapse very readily), by the presence of large amounts of mucus and by *oedema* (excess of tissue fluid) of the mucosa. In a normal person, air can be moved in and out of the lungs quickly, as shown in the tracing obtained from a spirometer (Fig. 4.4). Inspiration and expiration are deep and rapid, air is drawn in quickly and expelled quickly. In the bronchitic, the amount of air drawn in and out of the lungs is reduced. Inspiration is quick, but expiration is slow and prolonged.

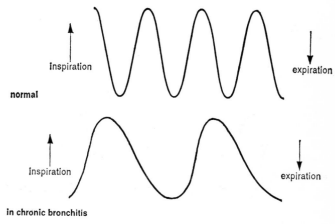

Inspiration

expiration

normal

Inspiration

expiration

in chronic bronchitis

Fig. 4.4 Spirometer tracings

Since some lung tissue is also destroyed by the formation of bullae, the forced vital capacity is lower than normal. Most noticeable is the fact that the amount of air which can be expired in one second (the FEV_1) is very much reduced. In the normal person at least 70 per cent of the total vital capacity can be expired in the first second, but in advanced chronic bronchitis this figure may be as low as 20 per cent. Another useful test is the peak expiratory flow rate using the Wright Peak Flow Meter (see p. 18). Instead of a normal maximum expiratory flow rate of at least 400 litres per minute, a chronic bronchitis adult may have a rate of only 60 litres per minute.

Because expiration is slow, the disease is also characterized by an increased concentration of carbon dioxide in the alveoli and in the blood. This increase can be measured by taking a sample of arterial blood and determining its degree of acidity, or by analysing a sample of alveolar air.

Treatment

A change of occupation may be necessary if the patient's present one involves exposure to dust and other irritants. In foggy weather, a smog mask may have to be worn if it is essential to be out of doors in such conditions, but it is better to remain in a warm room with the window shut. Crowded places of entertainment should be avoided when catarrhal infections are rife. Prophylactic immunization against influenza should be given in the late autumn, although this may not always be successful, since it is difficult to anticipate which type of influenza may be prevalent that winter.

Some patients benefit from taking a prophylactic broad-spectrum antibiotic, such as ampicillin or tetracycline, throughout the winter, but some physicians prefer vigorous early treatment of infections instead. Breathing exercises will help in relieving the patient's feeling of shortness of breath. Other general measures advised are reduction in weight (fat people are more prone to persistent respiratory infections), sleeping flat, and having the foot of the bed raised on blocks, to assist drainage of the bronchial tree (Fig. 4.5).

Prompt treatment of infection is essential. Such infection is first evident when the sputum becomes green or yellow instead of white or grey. The infecting organism in most cases is *Haemophilus in-*

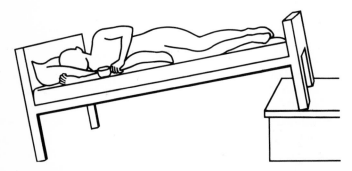

Fig. 4.5 The foot of the bed is raised to assist drainage of the bronchial tree

fluenzae, which is usually sensitive to tetraacycline (250 mg every 6 hours), amoxycillin (250 mg to 1 g every 6 hours) or septrin (2 tablets twice daily). Tetracycline is frequently used first as it is the cheapest. Both the clinical response and laboratory sensitivity tests can guide antibiotic therapy.

Cyanosis requires the administration of humidified oxygen, and portable oxygen can help by allowing the patient to move about between acute attacks. Pure oxygen, however, can be dangerous in chronic bronchitis.

In health, the respiratory centre in the brain responds to the concentration of carbon dioxide in the blood. But, in chronic bronchitis, the level of carbon dioxide in the blood is raised all the time, so the respiratory centre becomes insensitive to the action of carbon dioxide, and lack of oxygen is the only stimulus to breathing. If, therefore, too much oxygen is given to such patients, respiration slows down and may finally stop. The carbon dioxide level rises further, the patient becomes unconscious, and may die. Therefore, pure oxygen should not be given to a chronic bronchitic except under medical supervision.

Normal air contains 20 per cent oxygen, the rest being made up chiefly of nitrogen. Therefore, oxygen is usually given to a chronic bronchitic by means of a Venti mask (Fig. 4.6) or Edinburgh mask which gives a controlled percentage of oxygen. These masks help

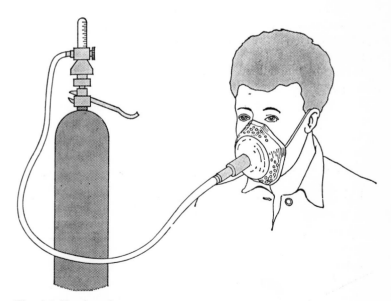

Fig. 4.6 Venti mask

the patient, but there is still a stimulus to respiration and the concentration of carbon dioxide does not rise to a dangerous level. It is best to start the patient needing oxygen with a mask providing 24 per cent oxygen. If the cyanosis persists and the patient does not become drowsy, a mask providing 28 per cent oxygen is given and, finally, one giving 30 per cent oxygen. If this percentage is not satisfactory, an oxygen tent can be used.

Tents give an oxygen concentration of about 40 per cent, but they should never be employed until use of the Venti mask has shown that the patient can take such a high concentration of oxygen without his respiratory rate decreasing or drowsiness occurring. When a Venti mask is not available, oxygen can be given via Tudor-Edwards spectacles or a nasal tube. When oxygen is prescribed to be administered by such a mask delivering a controlled flow it is essential to run the flow meter at the prescribed rate and no more. The practice of humidifying oxygen means that mucus secretions in the trachea and bronchi are not dried up and the sputum is therefore easier to expectorate – an important point for a weak and breathless patient. However the introduction of water into the circuit allows for any bacteria present in the tubing to multiply. For this reason nurses must ensure that all masks and tubings are disposed of as soon as they are no longer needed, to eliminate the risk of cross infection. All water containers for this purpose should be cleaned and refilled daily. Frequent observations should be made on the level of consciousness and depth of respiration of all patients with chronic bronchitis receiving oxygen. Medical aid should be sought if there is any evidence of drowsiness, because this means the respiratory centre in the brain is no longer being stimulated – coma and death will follow.

The cough is troublesome, particularly in the mornings; several sputum cartons will be required during the course of the day and the patient must be encouraged to expectorate. The aid of a physiotherapist may be enlisted.

Frequent attention to oral hygiene is necessary because of the foul sputum so mouth washes and refreshing drinks will be needed and adequate hydration facilitates the expectoration of sputum.

These patients are often undernourished because many of them live in difficult circumstances at home, frequently alone all day whilst other members of the family go out to work, or perhaps living entirely by themselves. This means they have to spend their limited financial resources on expensive convenience foods because they do not have the strength to shop and cook for themselves. The time in hospital may be used to establish a healthy eating pattern.

The pressure areas need particular care because many patients with chronic bronchitis have a degree of right sided cardiac failure due to their pulmonary congestion. Devitalised oedematous tissue breaks down readily at this stage in the illness and the sacrum is the dependant part, therefore the most oedematous.

As soon as the temperature subsides and the general condition improves the patient may sit out of bed and begin taking short walks.

Where cardiac failure develops, digoxin (0.25 mg) is given two or three times a day. A diuretic such as frusemide (40 mg daily) is also given with potassium supplements such as Slow K (1.2 g) three times a day. A fluid balance chart may be maintained but it is far more accurate to weigh the patient three times weekly on the same scales and in similar clothes each time, and a convenient place to record this is the temperature chart.

Smoking will of course have been forbidden during the time that O_2 was being administered. A change in routine and a period without nicotine may enable the patient to give up smoking and this should be encouraged if at all possible, because there is no doubt that smoking will further damage the lungs. Conversely an over-enthusiastic nurse is out of place because firstly a lot of damage has already been done; secondly, the quality of life of many of these patients is so poor that television and a packet of cigarettes is all they have, and it is cruel to deprive them of this pleasure. At this stage it is good to remember that an old man of 70 or 80 years has lived through two world wars and probably fought in one of them. His contribution to society has therefore been considerable and it is up to us to make his unfortunate circumstances as bearable as possible for him, particularly as he frequently attributes his lung condition to his wartime activities.

Normal sleeping patterns will be disturbed, partly because of the persistent coughing and partly because of the unaccustomed noise of a hospital ward at night. Night sedation may be prescribed but should only be given if essential and then not later than 1.00 a.m. Only drugs that do not supress the respiratory centre are used such as Mogadon 10 mgs. A common and sound practice is to suppress the cough with linctus codeine or linctus simplex and ensure mental and physical comfort. In most circumstances this is sufficient.

Wheezing can be treated with a number of different drugs: salbutamol (2 mg), ephedrine (30 mg), isoprenaline (10 mg) and aminophylline. To be really effective, aminophylline should be given intravenously in a dose of I g injected slowly. It has some action as a suppository, but only a very weak action when given by mouth.

Choline theophyllinate (200 mg) is a useful oral preparation or Phyllocontin 2 tablets twice daily.

If the bronchial secretions are thin and runny, tipping the bed and physiotherapy in the form of percussion of the chest may help. If the secretions are thick, *bronchial lavage* (surgical washing-out) may be necessary.

Many chronic bronchitis feel at their worst in the mornings. Later in the day, they are relatively comfortable and can get about and undertake some light work. Patients may claim that smoking a cigarette first thing in the morning helps them get their sputum up, but in reality this habit makes things worse and should be discouraged.

The teaching of breathing exercises can be helpful. It is important for the patient to concentrate on breathing out – frequently breathing exercises are wrongly associated with the idea of 'filling the chest with fresh air'.

There are two important points to stress in teaching breathing exercises: the abdominal muscles should be used to raise the diaphragm on expiration, and the chest and diaphragm should always work together. The procedure is as follows (Fig. 4.7):

a. The patient sits in an upright chair, with his back well supported. He should face a mirror.
b. He should relax and let his shoulders go slack, with his arms hanging by his side.
c. He should then place his fingernails against the lower edge of his rib cage, making sure that his shoulders are still relaxed and not pulled up.
d. He should then breathe out gently, without forcing the air out. As he exhales, he will feel his rib cage sink below his fingertips.
e. He should now breathe in gently and quietly, so that he feels the ribs lifting under his fingers.

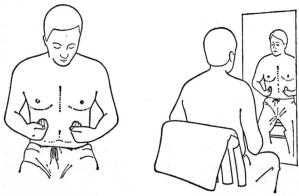

Fig. 4.7 Breathing exercises

This relaxed breathing is practised at a comfortable rate for approximately two or three minutes at least three times a day. Once the technique has been mastered, the mirror can be dispensed with. After further practice, the patient will not need to place his fingers on the chest wall. Eventually he will adopt this method of breathing and will continue it throughout the day without thinking.

Any other causes of shortness of breath which may be present will also be treated, e.g. blockage of the nose, wheezing, anaemia and early heart failure.

In very severe chronic bronchitics the amount of air inspired with each breath may drop as low as 250 ml as measured by a respirometer (a small instrument attached to a face mask). This volume fills only the nose, the pharynx, the trachea and major bronchi and none reaches the alveoli. A tracheostomy or tracheal intubation is then necessary so that this small amount of tidal air reaches the alveoli.

Broadly speaking intubation as a short term emergency measure may be simpler and quicker than tracheostomy. Nowadays the tubes used are non-reactory plastic e.g. portex and may be left in for up to four days; after this time subglottic friction may result in trauma producing stenosis of the trachea.

In cases which need airway assistance for longer than four days tracheostomy is the method of choice. It allows for the easy aspiration of secretions, reduces the dead space in ventilation and leaves the mouth free for feeding. The operation is usually carried out under light general anaesthesia and should be done before the patient's condition deteriorates too far. Minimal sedation is used preoperatively for this reason. The patient is put on the operating table with the head end slightly elevated and a small sandbag placed under the shoulders. The neck is extended with the neck held centrally. A transverse incision is made in the neck between the cricoid cartilage and the sternal notch, being careful to avoid the first two rings of the trachea. The deep fascia is cut vertically and the muscles over the front of the trachea retracted to each side. The isthmus of the thyroid is pushed upwards to expose the upper rings of the trachea. An opening is then made large enough to take the largest comfortably fitting tracheostomy tube. This may be either plastic or silver. If a cuff type is used this must not be overinflated. If a metal tube with a liner is used the liner must be changed and sterilised twice daily. Change of the tube must be made quickly since the ostium can stenose rapidly. The wound dressing should be changed daily and the skin surrounding the incision should be protected by barrier creams. Plastic tubes should be changed weekly and spare tubes available if the airway becomes blocked for any reason by dry secretions etc. When the time comes for removal of the tube, the tube opening is covered either by a valve or strapping to prevent an air leak and once the tube is removed the ostium closes rapidly of its own accord.

Both intubation and tracheostomy may be used in the I. T. U. of any hospital, particularly one dealing with chest diseases and chest surgery. A good supply of properly humidified air is required, since the problems of crusting and cleaning of the tubes are thereby reduced. There are a number of commercial humidifiers.

The best way to learn about intubation and tracheostomy is to endeavour to obtain permission to 'look in' on the work of an I. T. U as nothing can take the place of first hand practical instruction in the necessary procedures.

Summary comparing and contrasting tracheostomy and intubation

Intubation		Tracheostomy	
Advantages	Disadvantages	Advantages	Disadvantages
Simplicity	Experts required in constant attention	After operation is carried out can be looked after by nursing staff	It is an operation with dangers
Speed	Temporary (up to 4 days)	Can be permanent	Surgical shock
No scar			Scarring
No anaesthetic	Difficult to aspirate infections and crusts	Ease of aspiration of secretions	
	Discomfort in swallowing	Inner tube easily cleared	
	Stenosis after too long		

Tracheostomy

If a tracheostomy is performed the skills of the nurse are paramount in ensuring the patient's comfort and tranquility because he cannot communicate verbally. If time permits, and sometimes it does not, an explanation of the meaning and purpose of the procedure should be given to both patient and next of kin, and an assurance that he will have a nurse in attendance all the time the emergency lasts.

The room will be prepared with:

1. Suction equipment and a supply of sterile catheters
2. Oxygen
3. Ventilator with adaptor for the tracheostomy tubes
4. A selection of spare tracheostomy tubes
5. Tracheal dilators
6. Tape for tying the tube in position
7. Sterile gauze for dressings
8. Syringe gauze for dressings
8. Syringe for inflating the cuff
9. Humidifier or nebulizer
10. Observation chart

All unnecessary furniture should be moved from the area.

The observation chart will be maintained to monitor:

Temperature, pulse respiration
Blood pressure
Colour
Condition of skin
Level of consciousness
If used, the ventilator will be set to a pre-determined volume and tidal volume and pressure will be recorded.

By introducing a tracheostomy tube the dead space has been reduced but there are two other factors to prevent adequate ventilation. They are:

1. Contractions of smooth muscle causing diminution in the size of the lumen of the bronchioles
2. Copious sticky secretions which cannot be expectorated efficiently because the patient cannot build up any pressure of air in the trachea, even if he feels the need to cough. The effectiveness of the cough has been reduced because of the tarcheostomy and it is therefore necessary to assist the removal of secretions by suction

The procedure for aspiration of a tracheostomy tube varies from one centre to another but the general principles are the same.

It is important not to introduce infection. Some authorities advocate the use of sterile gloves to this end. Others do not. The cuff must be deflated, the sterile catheter moistened in sterile saline or water and gently introduced into the trachea – not until then is negative pressure applied and the catheter rotated until the airway is clear.

Frantic jerking up and down achieves very little except damage to the lining of the trachea. The whole procedure should take no more than 10–15 seconds. If it must be repeated there must be an interval of two minutes in order for the patient to settle down to a quiet respiratory rhythm again. It should be remembered that suction removes O_2 as well as secretions and it may be necessary to increase the oxygen supply after suction is performed in order to avoid hypoxia.

If the secretions are very sticky and difficult to dislodge distilled water may be instilled in measured quantities immediately before suction.

The irritation of the mucosal lining by the catheter may stimulate coughing – material expectorated in this way must be swiftly but gently wiped away with gauze or Kleenex before it is sucked back with the next inspiration. The cuff is reflated: the catheter thrown away: a specimen of sputum is sent for culture and bacterial sensitivity.

Care of the tube and wound

Tubes in common use today are made of synthetic material and do not have an inner lining, but they do have a cuff which must be inflated if a ventilator is used. They need to be changed every 24 hours. The surrounding skin is kept dry and free from secretions. A keyhole dressing is applied.

A note pad and pencil is provided for the patient to communicate. It is better if the care of this patient can be the responsibility of a limited number of nurses who quickly become very astute in assessing the needs without the necessity of the patient writing everything. As the days pass the patient will be taught to put his clean finger over the tube enabling him to speak short sentences.

When it becomes unnecessary to apply suction each hour the cuff should still be deflated for a few minutes at regular intervals in order to avoid ulceration of the wall of the trachea.

The patient will be weaned off the ventilator by switching it off for increasing periods during the day until he is able to breathe without it for several hours. The timing of this operation is clearly decided by the medical staff. It should be done before the patient settles into a state of mind in which he is dependant on it.

The large tracheostomy tube is replaced by a smaller silver tube when the use of the ventilator is discontinued. After a few days the tube may be removed and a Vaseline gauze dressing applied. The hole will close in about forty-eight hours.

There is a very understandable fear that swallowing is impossible whilst a tracheostomy tube is in situ. The wise nurse will give her patients sips of water very quickly after the operation to avoid this problem, remembering the close relationship between oesophagus and trachea. It is usual for a broad spectrum antibiotic to be prescribed as a prophylactic measure against infection whilst a tracheostomy tube is in situ.

Considerable psychological support will be required because the function of the glottis and the larynx is lost and therefore it is difficult to express any emotional feelings. Patients are unable to differentiate between night and day because the rituals of turning, coughing and suction continue during 24 hours.

Clinical observation of the patient is of prime importance. The type of respiration; laboured, with the uses of the accessory muscles of respiration, the excursion of the thorax, the colour and condition of the skin and changes in character of the mucus secretions should all be recorded and reported.

By listening the nurse will be aware of changes in respiration, the existence of secretions in the respiratory tract and any changes which may occur as a result of alterations in respiratory or cardiac systems.

Asthma

Asthma is a disease characterized by recurrent attacks of wheezing which occur mainly or entirely during expiration. These are due to spasm of the bronchial muscles and oedema of the bronchial mucosa. Typically, asthma occurs in bouts, and the sufferer feels perfectly normal in the intervals between. In some cases the wheeze becomes almost continuous, although a variability in the degree of airway obstruction can be observed.

Asthma is a very common disease which can occur in any age group. There seems to be a hereditary constitutional factor which makes some people liable to wheeze, and this wheeze can be triggered in a number of ways.

Two types of asthma are recognized:

a. *extrinsic asthma*: having its origins in external agents to which the sufferer becomes sensitive;

b. *intrinsic asthma*: developing in middle age or later adult life and unrelated to known external allergens.

Extrinsic asthma

A condition of unusual or exaggerated susceptibility to a substance which is harmless in similar amounts to the majority of people is known as an *allergy*. The substances (*allergens*) responsible for asthma in susceptible people include pollens, moulds, feathers, wool, dog and cat hair, house dust, flour, agricultural fertilizers, animal foodstuffs, eggs, shellfish, nuts, chocolate and drugs such as aspirin. Of all these allergens, house dust and pollen are probably the most important. House dust has recently been shown to contain a tiny mite called *Dermatophagoides*, and it is probably the inhalation of the faeces from these tiny creatures that provokes asthmatic attacks. Another important cause of asthma is exposure to substances met at work. Thus asthma can be caused in some people by working with platinum salts, solderers can become sensitive to epoxy resins in the flux, carpenters to the dust from some hard woods and laboratory attendants to the urine and faeces from experimental animals. Initial contact with any of these allergens is said to 'sensitize' the patient, so that his body produces antibodies to it. At the next exposure to the allergen, a violent reaction takes place in the lungs and the bronchi. The mucosa which lines the bronchi becomes swollen and the bronchial muscles go into spasm, so that the lumen of the tubes is reduced in size. In addition, the bronchial glands secrete thick, sticky mucus which creates further obstruction.

This violent reaction is due to the release of *histamine* (a chemical which stimulates smooth muscle, dilates the capillaries and allows their walls to leak fluid into the tissues) and also of another substance called *slow reacting substance*.

Intrinsic asthma

Most cases of intrinsic asthma are associated with infection, mainly chronic inflammation of the bronchi. The allergic component of the disease is minimal or non-existent.

Even when the asthmatic pattern of reaction to extrinsic agents or infection has become established, attacks may be precipitated by many other causes such as emotional stress, physical exertion, changes in temperature or humidity, irritant fumes or smoke.

Whatever the cause, the result is a narrowing of the bronchial air passages and this, combined with obstruction by mucus, hinders the ventilation of the lungs. Increased respiratory effort, with use of the accessory muscles of respiration, increases the efficiency of inspiration more than that of expiration so that the lungs become progressively distended with air as the attack proceeds. This produces an acute emphysema. Aeration of the blood becomes impaired and in severe attacks cyanosis occurs.

The attack subsides as the constricted bronchi gradually widen. Once the obstruction is relieved, the lungs rapidly return to normal. Here, asthma differs from both chronic bronchitis and emphysema where the condition of the lungs never returns to normal between exacerbations.

Symptoms

Asthma usually occurs in periodic spasms, and the patient may feel quite well between attacks. It may occur at only one time of the year if the patient is allergic to grass pollen; it may occur only at night if house dust in the bedroom provokes attacks. The onset of an attack is usually sudden: the patient complains of a feeling of suffocation and pressure on the chest, he starts to breathe faster and faster, and there is an audible wheeze with each expiration. He is usually distressed, and has to sit bolt upright to make breathing easier. The accessory muscles of respiration are used in an attempt to force air through the narrowed bronchioles. The chest becomes hyper-expanded and there may be cyanosis. At the end of the attack, the asthmatic may bring up large amounts of thick mucoid sputum.

Most attacks subside within an hour or two. In some cases, an acute attack may persist for some days. The patient is then said to be in *status asthmaticus*, and the resulting fatigue and loss of sleep cause severe debilitation, and can threaten life because of the increasing obstruction of the smaller airways by tenacious mucus plugs. A number of patients remain in a chronic state of mild asthma, especially during the hay fever season. Although they appear normal at rest, they suffer from shortness of breath and wheezing on any exertion or emotional excitement.

Diagnosis

This is usually easy if the patient is seen in an acute attack. The history of asthma or other allergic disorders in other members of the family is valuable supporting evidence. The blood usually shows an increase in the eosinophil white cells (white cells containing granules readily stained by eosin) above the maximum level of 400 per mm^3 of blood, and these cells may also be found in the sputum.

A chest X-ray between attacks shows no abnormality, but is useful in excluding other diseases. During an attack the lung fields appear distended, with depression of the dome of the diaphragm, elevation of the ribs and some increase in the lung markings.

Treatment

There are three aspects of this:

a. Symptomatic relief of the attack
b. Control of specific causative factors
c. General care of the patient

Symptomatic relief of the attack

The measures used depend upon the severity of the attacks. In mild cases bronchodilators such as Salbutamol (Ventolin) 2 or 4 mg thrice daily by mouth, Phyllocontin 2 tablets twice daily or Aminophyllin suppositories, one twice daily, may be sufficient.

Where these fail bronchodilators given by inhalation are often effective, since then the drugs reach the bronchi directly. Salbutamol (Ventolin), Terbutaline (Bricanyl) and Adrenalin (Medihaler Iso) can be given in this form. A standard metered dose of the drug is delivered in the form of an aerosol by means of a pressurised dispenser. Bronchoconstriction is usually relieved for up to three or four hours. There is reason to believe that over-use of these aerosols can lead to death in a number of patients due to cardiac toxicity in a patient who is already short of oxygen. These inhalers should not, therefore, be used more than six times in twenty four hours and if the patient is not getting relief he must call his doctor for a change in his treatment.

It is important that these aerosols are used correctly. The patient should sit relaxed in a chair. He should breath out as far as possible, then open his mouth and deliver the aerosol dose into the mouth, at the same time breathing in as far as possible. He should then hold his breath as long as possible and then let the air out of his lungs as slowly as possible. This procedure should then be repeated with a second puff from the aerosol.

A valuable combination of aerosols is that of Ventolin or Bricanyl with Becotide. Becotide is a form of cortisone which acts locally on the bronchial mucosa with none of the side effects resulting from taking cortisone preparations by mouth since little is absorbed from an aerosol into the general circulation. Occasionally thrush can develop in the mouth from its use and this can be controlled by sucking Nystatin lozenges. The Ventolin or Bricanyl is used first to dilate the bronchi and is followed ten minutes later with two puffs from the Becotide inhaler.

Such a combination of inhalers used four to six times a day can keep a person free of asthma and the dose can then be reduced over a period of weeks. If the patient can be kept free of asthma for a long time the attacks frequently die out.

Sodium Cromoglycate (Intal) is a prophylactic agent which prevents the release of substances in the lung which cause bronchoconstriction. The drug has to be taken regularly as an inhaled powder in a special spinhaler. Initially four capsules a day are taken but the number may be reduced subsequently. It is particularly effective in asthma produced by exertion. It must be emphasised to the patient that the drug only prevents attacks so that the inhalations must be continued even if no attacks of asthma are occurring. The drug is useless in an attack of asthma.

In cases where an attack of asthma occurs in spite of using inhalers, treatment by injection then becomes necessary. Aminophyllin 250–500 mg or Ventolin 250 micrograms given slowly intravenously may relieve an attack. This can be followed by giving corticosteroids by mouth. Because of the severe side effects which can result from prolonged use of these drugs the criterion for use must be that the dangers from prolonged use are less dangerous than the disease itself which may be threatening life.

In some patients normal activities may be impossible without the long term administration of these drugs. Treatment is usually started with 40 mg of Prednisolone daily reducing to a maintainance dose which is usually 10 mg daily. In children oral corticosteroids often stunt growth and it is usual, therefore, to use injections of A.C.T.H. Treatment is usually started with 40 units intramuscularly daily. Once the respiratory function has returned to normal the interval between injections may be slowly lengthened up to a week.

An intravenous drip of sodium bicarbonate is required to correct acidosis. A drip is also set up of 500 mg aminophyllin or 500 micrograms Ventolin in 500 ml glucose saline is given over a period of four hours. These doses are repeated as often as necessary. In addition 1,000 mg of hydrocortisone may be given into the drip over a period of twelve hours. Once the drip has been terminated treatment is continued either with oral steroids or with 0.5% Salbutamol given by intermittent positive pressure ventilation with a Bird or Barnet respirator.

Sedatives are often required since the patient may be in desperate need of sleep. Morphine and barbiturates are contra-indicated since they depress respiration. Valium (Diazepam) 10 mg or Phenergan (Promethazine Hydrochloride) 25–50 mg are useful drugs.

If the above measures are not successful the patient becomes weaker and cyanosed because only small amounts of air are taken in with each breath and this amount may be insufficient to reach the alveoli and merely passes up and down the main bronchi. In such cases intubation or a tracheostomy is necessary. By this manoeuvre the nose, pharynx and larynx are by-passed and so the small amount of air which is being breathed in has more chance of reaching the alveoli and oxygenating the blood. A tracheostomy has the advantage that a small rubber suction tube can be passed through the tracheostomy tube and mucus sucked out of the bronchial tree. This is especially valuable in children in whom the small bronchi are easily blocked. If necessary a mechanical ventilator can also be attached to the endotracheal tube.

The popular mechanical ventilator is one that is volume cycled (Cape or Smith-Clar) in which 6–8 litres of gas is given per minute at a breathing rate below 20 per minute.

Oxygen given by machine must be humidified, preferably with a temperature controlled heated humidifier, since the humidifying action of the upper respiratory tract is cut out by intubation. Patients on a respirator must be watched to make sure that the chest is moving and for cyanosis. Pulse rate, blood pressure, fluid intake and urine output must be measured and charted for assessing progress. Weaning from the machine is gradual and started during the day. Regular measurement of blood gases help in assessing the returning efficiency of the respiratory system as well as the pulse rate, beathing rate and tidal volume.

Nursing care

The aim of nursing care of a patient in an acute attack of asthma is to relieve the bronchial spasm and to prevent its recurrence.

Firstly the cause must be determined by adequate investigation and observation. If an allergen is responsible it is relatively easy in some cases to remove it from the patient's environment. It is quite impossible to remove stress from life and at best we can only hope to reduce it and perhaps enable people to regard their anxieties in a more philosophical way. Infection will be treated with antibiotics.

A dyspoenic, wheezy patient with thick tenacious sputum needs to be sat up in bed leaning on a bedtable. This enables her/him to use the accessory muscles or respiration. The bedtable should be covered by a pillow to protect the patient from the sharp edges. The nurse should remain in attendance because there is a marked tendency to panic in a situation where the patient is exhausted with lack of sleep and the tremendous effort that is required to breathe.

A 15–30 minute pulse chart may be indicated because there are changes in the systemic and pulmonary circulations. Tachycardia is common, a rising pulse rate with changing volume will alert the nurse to the possibility of cardiac arrest. Pulsus paradoxus describes a situation where alterations in intra thoracic pressure interferes with the pumping action of the heart and during inspiration the radial beat can be felt to be much weaker than on expiration. This is another danger sign. The blood pressure should be monitored because the nurse must be aware of any fall in cardiac output.

The prolonged dyspnoea causes a reduction in arterial oxygen and confusion and restlessness follows, so blood gas analysis must be done and oxygen administered with a polymask or B.L.B. mask and it should be saturated with water vapour. (In the presence of chronic bronchitis and/or emphysema a ventimask delivering 24% solution of oxygen will be prescribed in the first instance.)

Control of specific factors

A detailed history from the patient may show that he is sensitive to grass pollens, to house dust, to certain foods or to a drug such as aspirin. The patient's occupation may also be important since this may expose him to known allergens. Hobbies may involve the keeping of budgerigars, pigeons, dogs or other pets.

When any allergen is suspected it should, as far as possible, be removed from the patient's environment. Thus, feather pillows may need to be replaced by foam and woollen blankets by cotton ones. The mattress may need to be placed in a polythene bag. Pets may have to be removed. The bedroom may need an intensive cleaning with complete removal of curtains, carpets, cushions and anything else that could harbour the house-dust mite.

Further information about a patient's sensitivities can be obtained from skin testing. Solutions of various allergens are commercially available. In the prick test, a small drop of the solution is placed on the forearm and a needle is then pricked through the drop into the patient's skin. A control test is carried out on the other arm. The results are read ten minutes later and compared with the result given by the control solution. A positive reaction is shown by the presence of a weal, caused by outpouring of fluid

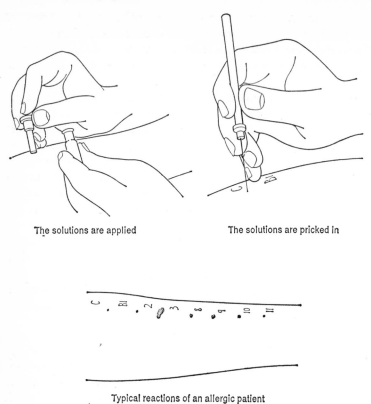

The solutions are applied   The solutions are pricked in

Typical reactions of an allergic patient

Fig. 4.8 Skin testing

from the capillaries into the skin (Fig. 4.8). The intensity of the reaction is recorded by measuring the diameter of the weal in millimetres.

Unfortunately, skin tests are useful in only a small proportion of asthma cases. Where there is an obvious causal relationship with an allergen, however, the sensitivity of the patient to this allergen can sometimes be reduced by a course of injections of a solution of the offending substance.

In general, treatment begins with injections of no more than twice the amount of antigen injected in the intracutaneous test, increasing weekly and aiming to reach a dose approximately 500 times the initial one. The injections are given subcutaneously on the lateral aspect of the upper arm. Adrenaline 1:1000 solution is kept at hand in case of an excessive reaction. On the first occasion, the patient should be kept under observation for 20 minutes after the injection. A course of water-soluble antigens requires about 20 injections. If alum-precipitated compounds are used, then only 6 to 8 injections are needed. Usually one course is sufficient, but in some patients up to three courses may be necessary to relieve the asthma.

If attacks occur during the winter, the cause may be an infection, particularly if the sputum is persistently green or yellow. In children, especially, attacks are often preceded by a cold, although both extrinsic allergens and infections may be important. The presence of chronic sinusitis or nasal polyps suggests an infective factor. The persistence of asthma for a few days after admission to hospital, when contact with many allergens is broken, also suggests this. If the temperature is raised at the start of an attack, this also indicates that infection may be present.

Infective asthma should be vigorously treated with antibiotics. Asthmatic patients are particularly susceptible to severe penicillin reactions, so this drug is usually withheld. Adequate drainage of infected para-nasal sinuses should be carried out and nasal polyps removed.

Intravenous therapy. If the condition warrants intravenous therapy the routine care of the equipment will be the responsibility of the nurse. The drugs added to the solutions must always be checked, according to local policy, by two trained nurses. The limb in which the cannula or needle is inserted must be supported and kept warm to prevent the vein going into spasm. Observation must be made at intervals to ensure that it is running at the prescribed rate and is not going into the tissues.

General care of the patient

This involves avoidance of the secondary factors liable to aggravate asthma, e.g. extremes of cold and humidity, and smoking. Breathing exercises from a trained physiotherapist are valuable in preventing chest deformities and postural defects. Adequate relaxation, holidays and avoidance of overwork are essential.

Emotional factors are common in children, especially if the mother is over-anxious and if the child gains advantages from having asthma attacks.

In many cases eradication of the cause is impossible, and persistent wheezing becomes very disabling so that bronchodilators have to be used for long periods.

Prognosis

Asthma is a chronic, relapsing disease. It is common in children, but clears up in about 30 per cent of patients by adolescence; it sometimes recurs around the age of twenty. In adults the disease tends to be progressive, attacks becoming more frequent and prolonged. Infective asthma in the elderly usually becomes chronic and the illness is similar to chronic bronchitis.

Death used to be a relatively rare outcome of an attack of asthma but this is no longer true, especially in children. It is believed that the increase in deaths has been due to the over-use of pressurized aerosols and a reluctance to use steroids in adequate dosage. A greater awareness by doctors and patients of this has saved a number of lives.

Foreign bodies in the air passages

The aspiration of foreign bodies into the trachea and bronchi is a frequent cause of pulmonary disease which may be overlooked unless a careful history is taken. When aspiration occurs, there is a fit of coughing which passes off when the foreign body reaches the smaller bronchi. There is then a silent interval until cough and sputum develop. At this stage the previous coughing bout is often forgotten and all that can be found is a collapsed, infected lobe.

Carelessness is responsible for most foreign bodies being in the respiratory tract. Workmen and housewives frequently hold nails or pins in their mouths and these are aspirated if the person is startled or makes a sudden movement. A filling or broken tooth can be aspirated during dental operations. Young children frequently put small toys in their mouth and then swallow or aspirate them. Peanuts may be inhaled, and can cause quite a severe inflammatory reaction in the bronchi. Rapid eating, especially after drinking a great deal of alcohol, is a common cause of food being aspirated into the respiratory tract.

A large foreign body that completely obstructs the trachea can cause death from suffocation. A small foreign body may jam in the vocal cords. This results in reflex closure of the larynx, with immediate death. If a foreign body passes into the bronchi, the symptoms may be very slight, especially if the object is small. Often, however, there is choking, gasping, severe cough, shortness of breath and cyanosis. A loud wheeze may be audible to someone standing near the patient.

After a time, the symptoms may clear completely and, days or

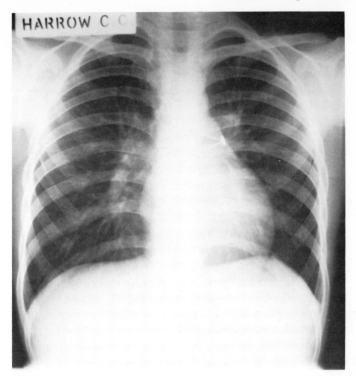

Fig. 4.9 X-ray showing paper clip in left main bronchus

weeks later, cough, sputum and a raised temperature appear. A chest X-ray usually shows partial collapse of the lung, due to obstruction of the supplying bronchus. Frequently the foreign body cannot be seen on X-ray, even when it is a highly radio-opaque such as a tooth. Thus, diagnosis has to be made on the history.

Unless the foreign body is removed, the outlook is poor. Bronchoscopy must be carried out as soon as possible. Even when the foreign body has been present in the lung for some months, its removal can lead to a complete recovery of the damaged lung. After removal, therefore, observation is carried out for a period before the doctor decides that the affected portion of lung should be removed.

Lung abscess

The formation of an abscess in the lung means that there has been rapid death of part of the lung tissue. Most lung abscesses start with bronchial obstruction leading to collapse of part of the lung, which is then invaded by virulent organisms. The usual underlying causes are:

a. *Aspiration*: septic material may be inhaled during an operation on the upper respiratory tract or during a dental operation.
b. *Embolic*: infected material can reach the lungs from blood clots coming from a septic area of the body. The blood in the veins near such an area clots and becomes invaded by bacteria (*septic thrombophlebitis*) and parts of the clot can work loose and be carried in the blood stream to the lungs. Such abscesses are usually small and multiple, and can be found in any part of the lung.
c. *Post-pneumonic*: this is especially likely when pneumonia occurs in debilitated, old people. Chronic small abscesses result.
d. *Bronchogenic*: infection occurs round a foreign body in a bronchus or around a bronchial carcinoma or other type of bronchial stenosis.
e. *Traumatic*: in chest wounds, a bullet or a piece of clothing may become lodged in the lung. Infection round this leads to abscess formation. Fractured ribs may cause a blood clot to form in the lung tissue, and subsequent infection of this clot leads to the formation of an abscess.
f. *Infected cysts*: both hydatid and congenital cysts in the lung (*bronchogenic cysts*) can become infected during a minor respiratory infection such as a cold, and abscess formation may result. This is rare.
g. *Trans-diaphragmatic*: a subphrenic abscess or an abscess in the liver may rupture through the diaphragm and give rise to an abscess in the right lower lobe of the lung.

The onset of a lung abscess is usually acute, with the patient complaining of fever, shivering, sweating, malaise and loss of appetite. There is an irritating cough with the production of a little mucus. Acute pain will be felt if the pleura is involved. In about three-quarters of the cases, the sputum is stained with blood.

After some days the abscess ruptures into a bronchus and the patient coughs up large amounts of foul-smelling purulent sputum. The temperature then falls and the patient feels much better, although he still coughs and expectorates. In the acute phase, a chest X-ray shows an irregular shadow in one part of the lung with a large, ragged cavity containing a fluid level (Fig. 4.10). The complications of a lung abscess include pleurisy, empyema, pyopneumothorax, brain abscess and septicaemia.

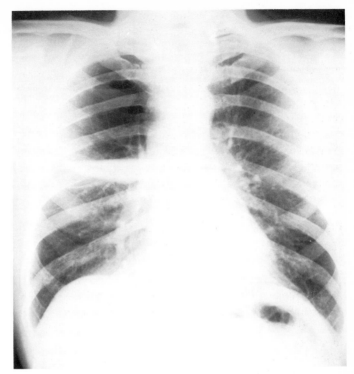

Fig. 4.10 An X-ray showing lung abscess

Treatment

Treatment consists of the administration of an antibiotic and post-ural drainage. Regular sputum cultures are essential so that appropriate antibiotics can be given if new invading organisms appear during the course of treatment.

For postural drainage the patient is placed in such a position that the abscess is at the highest part of the chest, so that all the secre-tions produced by the abscess run into the bronchial tree and are coughed up. For an abscess in one lower lobe, the patient lies on his side with the affected side uppermost and the foot of the bed raised 45–50 cm. The middle lobe and lingula are drained by lying the patient flat on his back and raising the foot of the bed. Each up-per lobe may be drained by sitting the patient up and leaning him away from the affected side (Fig. 4.11).

With postural drainage and prolonged antibiotic treatment (often up to four weeks), the abscess cavity usually closes, leaving only a

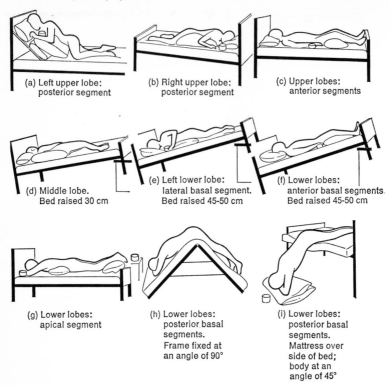

(a) Left upper lobe:
    posterior segment

(b) Right upper lobe:
    posterior segment

(c) Upper lobes:
    anterior segments

(d) Middle lobe.
    Bed raised 30 cm

(e) Left lower lobe:
    lateral basal segment.
    Bed raised 45-50 cm

(f) Lower lobes:
    anterior basal segments.
    Bed raised 45-50 cm

(g) Lower lobes:
    apical segment

(h) Lower lobes:
    posterior basal
    segments.
    Frame fixed at
    an angle of 90°

(i) Lower lobes:
    posterior basal
    segments.
    Mattress over
    side of bed;
    body at an
    angle of 45°

Fig. 4.11 Positions for postural drainage

small scar. Occasionally, the abscess cavity does not drain properly. In these cases the surgeon makes an incision through the lung into the abscess cavity and clears out the debris inside. A small drainage tube is then inserted into the cavity and through this a solution of the appropriate antibiotic is instilled every six hours. As the abscess cavity closes, the drainage tube is gradually shortened. The steady reduction in size of the cavity can be seen on the X-ray while the cavity is still large. When it is smaller, its size can be determined by running radio-opaque material down the drainage tube and taking an X-ray picture. Occasionally, the lobe containing the abscess cavity has to be resected.

Nursing care. All cases of lung abscess must be bronchoscoped after recovery to ensure that a bronchial carcinoma is not present as the underlying cause of the lung abscess.

The optimum postural drainage position must be maintained during the night as well as the day. This causes discomfort and the patient needs encouragement.

Frequent attention to oral hygiene is necessary because of the foul smelling sputum passing through the mouth.

In the event of external drainage becoming necessary dressings will be renewed twice daily under aseptic conditions.

Complications. Cerebral abscess will cause renewed fever, lethargy and a slowing of the pulse rate. Amyloid disease will cause waxy degeneration of tissue in some organs.

Five
Generalized diseases of the lung

Tuberculosis

It is said that between a half and one per cent of the world's population is coughing up tubercle bacilli. In some tropical countries tuberculosis is still one of the most prevalent diseases, but in the United Kingdom and many other temperate countries its incidence has fallen dramatically in the last thirty years.

Tuberculosis is caused by the microorganism *Mycobacterium tuberculosis*, which is found in the sputum and discharges of tuberculous patients. The bacillus is a slender, straight or slightly curved rod-shaped organism 2.5 to 3.5 μm long (Fig. 5.1). It is non-mobile and there are four types: human, bovine, avian and piscine, so-called because of their occurrence in men, cattle, birds and fishes respectively. The human and bovine types can infect man, but infection by the latter type is now rare in Western countries, due to the large scale pasteurisation of milk.

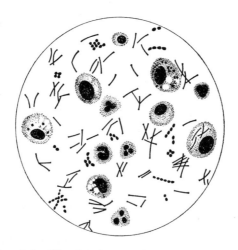

Fig. 5.1 Tubercle bacilli – showing as rods amongst the sputum cells

The tubercle bacillus is difficult to stain when it is being sought in sputum. The nurse must ensure that the specimen sent to the laboratory is sputum and not saliva. The sputum is spread on a microscope slide, dried and then stained with a dye called *carbolfuchsin*. Since the tubercle bacillus has a wax envelope, it will not take up the carbolfuchsin unless the dye on the slide is heated. Once the tubercle bacillus has taken up this red stain, it cannot be removed by washing with acid or alcohol. For this reason, the tubercle bacillus is often referred to as an *acid-fast bacillus* (*AFB*).

Culture of the organism is also difficult. It does not grow on ordinary media but requires special media enriched with egg yolk and potato starch (*Löwenstein's medium*). Even on this medium, growth is slow and a positive culture takes six to eight weeks to obtain.

The tubercle bacillus thrives in damp, ill-ventilated places. It is rapidly destroyed by direct sunlight, but can withstand 5 per cent Lysol for fifteen minutes, dry heat at 100 °C (212 °F) for twenty minutes or moist heat at 60 °C (140 °F) for twenty minutes. It can resist ordinary cold, it is not destroyed by the acid in gastric juice and it can live in house dust for several days. It is, however, killed in the process of pasteurization of milk, in which the milk is heated to 71 °C (161 °F) for fifteen seconds and then cooled rapidly to 4 °C (40 °F).

Once a person has become infected, the consequences depend upon the infecting dose and the patient's resistance. Natural resistance varies in different countries, depending on local conditions. People living in small communities may be very susceptible, particularly if these communities were once isolated and have been brought into contact with infectious cases only recently, as transport has improved.

Whether active disease follows on infection depends not only on the native resistence but also on poor ventilation, absence of sunlight, and inadequate nutrition. Certain occupations are very prone to the disease, e.g. sand-blasting, grinding, mining and the preparation of asbestos products.

Infection

The tubercle bacillus can gain entry to the body in three ways:

a. Inhalation. Today the inhalation of air containing tubercle bacilli is the most important means of acquiring tuberculous infection. The bacilli may be transported in droplets of saliva or sputum, but infection can also occur from inhalation of particles of dust laden with the microorganism because of the peculiar resistance of the bacilli to drying or exposure.

b. Ingestion. The tubercle bacilli may enter the mouth and pharynx by direct or indirect contact with infected material. Tuberculous food handlers, for example, may deposit organisms on food or eating utensils. This will lead to infection in the tonsil or in the abdomen. Kissing may also transmit infection. Dogs are susceptible to the tubercle bacillus, and can occasionally transmit the disease to humans.

c. Penetration through the skin. This is mainly an occupational hazard of men working in slaughter houses and of pathologists, who may become infected by cutting themselves while doing post-mortems or while working with germ cultures.

The disease is not inherited, although the degree of resistance which a person has is partly inherited from the parents. The sources of infection are:

1. Infectious patients. This is by far the commonest cause. The use of Mass Radiography Units, which concentrate on X-raying apparently healthy people, has shown that a substantial number of apparently healthy adults are suffering from active tuberculosis. About half of these have a positive sputum (in other words, the tubercle bacillus can be isolated from their sputum). Yet a great many of these people are unaware that they have anything wrong with them. A smaller problem is the uncooperative infectious patient who discharges himself from hospital against medical advice.

2. Food. The most important food is milk, but this source of infection has almost been abolished in most Western countries by pasteurization and the tuberculin testing of cattle. Infection is usually with the bovine bacillus which tends to affect the lymph glands, bones and joints, rather than the lungs.

Once the tubercle bacilli have entered the tissues, the response is either exudative or protective. An *exudative* lesion (Fig. 5.2) tends to occur when large doses of highly virulent organisms infect loose tissue structures such as the lungs. The white cells surround the tubercle bacillus and infiltrate the alveoli. After a variable period of time, this pneumonic type of lesion may be absorbed or it may *caseate* (a process in which all the cells are killed and acquire a cheesy

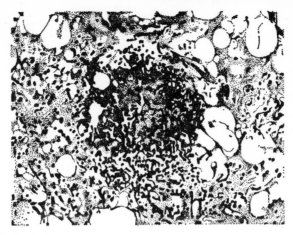

Fig. 5.2 Exudative response

consistency). These caseous areas may be gradually replaced by fibrosis and calcification.

Protective reactions (Fig. 5.3) are commonly observed when small doses of tubercle bacilli of low virulence infect firm tissue structures. The protective lesion or tubercle, from which the disease gets its name, involves the growth of new granulation tissues which push the normal tissue aside. Later a fibrous capsule surrounds the tubercle and eventually calcification of these small tubercles may occur.

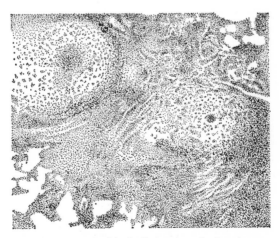

Fig. 5.3 Protective response with the formation of tubercles

Infection of the human body with tuberculosis occurs in three stages:

The primary complex

In a person who is infected with tuberculosis for the first time, a small area of inflammation occurs at the point where the tubercle bacilli lodge after entry to the body, and the glands draining this area become considerably enlarged. This primary focus is known as a *Parrot–Ghon focus* and occurs most commonly in the lung. The pulmonary lesion is usually very small, but the enlargement of the glands in the root of the lung is very obvious on a chest X-ray (Fig. 5.4). In the majority of cases the primary complex undergoes spontaneous healing and, eventually, calcification occurs. In a small percentage of cases, the pulmonary lesion enlarges and cavitation occurs as the cells in the centre of the area of inflammation are killed, become fluid and are coughed up.

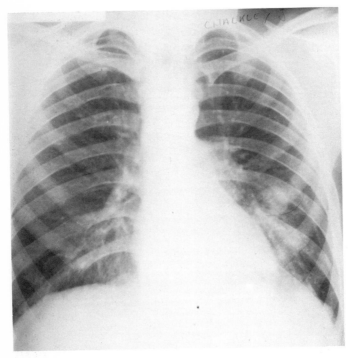

Fig. 5.4 An X-ray showing enlargement of the glands in the root of the lung

When the tubercle bacilli are ingested through the mouth, the primary focus usually occurs in the tonsil, with enlargement of the glands in the neck. If the tubercle bacilli pass through the pharynx and stomach and enter the small intestine, the primary lesion is formed in the *Peyer's patches* (small areas of lymphoid tissue present in the intestinal mucosa). The lymph glands in the abdomen will then become enlarged.

Blood spread

Not all the tubercle bacilli are trapped by the lymph nodes. Some pass along the lymphatics to the lymphatic duct and into the blood stream. Spread via the blood is believed to occur in all cases of primary tuberculosis. In those who have poor resistance, acute disease appears within about three months of the primary infection. Such acute manifestations may be of two types: in *miliary tuberculosis* (Fig. 5.5), small tubercles the size of millet seeds are formed in various organs of the body such as the lungs, the brain and kid-

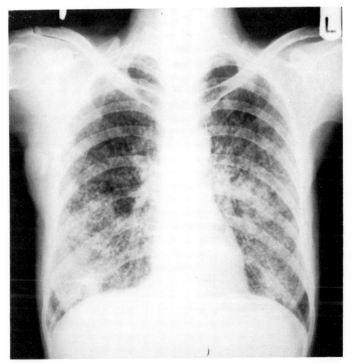

Fig. 5.5 Miliary tuberculosis

neys; in *tuberculous meningitis*, the membranes covering the brain become infected.

Nowadays, both of these conditions are rare in Western countries. In some people there are no acute manifestations but, two to three years after the primary infection, disease develops in the kidneys, bones, joints or in the apices of the lungs.

Adult-type disease

The third and final stage of this disease is adult, bronchogenic tuberculosis. This occurs three to five years after the primary infection has occurred, although its appearance may be deferred for a longer period. The fibrous tissue enveloping the tubercle bacilli at the top of the lung breaks down and softens, and the disease then spreads through the lung (Fig. 5.6). When a fairly large area has become involved, softening occurs, with the formation of cavities. This is dangerous, since the walls of these cavities are always teeming with tubercle bacilli. As a result, the sputum will be full of the bacilli. This sputum may well be coughed up but, especially if the

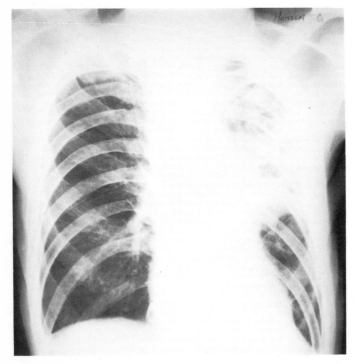

Fig. 5.6 Adult-type tuberculosis

patient is asleep, the sputum may fail to reach the mouth and instead will drop back into a fresh part of the lung and lead to the development of further disease.

Age is an important factor in determining what will happen when a person is infected with the tubercle bacilli. If the patient is a baby, a primary focus in the lungs is especially liable to progress, so miliary tuberculosis or meningitis is more likely than it would be in an adult. Between the ages of five and ten, a primary tuberculous infection is relatively benign and may be unsuspected: the child may complain of tiredness and be off his food for seven to ten days (symptoms which are extremely common in young children). Unless he has a chest X-ray, the cause of his symptoms will not be diagnosed. In men over the age of forty-five, healed tuberculous lesions are liable to break down. Thus, many authorities say that men of this age are unlikely to develop active tuberculosis unless their chest X-rays show evidence of old, healed tuberculous disease.

Diagnosis

The symptoms of tuberculosis can mimic almost any other disease, and many cases which have been puzzling are only diagnosed at a post-mortem examination. Suspicious symptoms include:

a. Coughing up blood (haemoptysis)
b. Shortness of breath
c. Severe pain due to the onset of pleurisy
d. Symptoms like those of lobar pneumonia (see p. 33), but with no response to antibiotics
e. Tiredness
f. Unexplained weight loss
g. Persistent cough
h. Recurrent fever and sweating at night.

In children, symptoms are rarely respiratory in origin. They are more likely to complain of malaise, tiredness and loss of appetite.

Complications include: tuberculous laryngitis, ulceration of the small intestine, spontaneous pneumothorax, pleural effusion, infection of bones, joints, glands, skin and kidney.

Pulmonary tuberculosis is now mainly diagnosed through radiological examination of the chest. Full confirmation of the diagnosis is made by the isolation of the tubercle bacilli, usually from a smear of sputum and (six weeks later) by a positive culture. When no sputum can be produced, the material obtained by gastric lavage can be cultured or a laryngeal swab used.

Gastric lavage

The patient is given no food or drink after 22.00 hours the previous evening. The contents of the stomach are removed as soon as possible after waking in the morning. This time is chosen because the material is not then mixed with food, and also because gastric peristalsis is diminished during the night, so that the more viscid contents tend to collect in the stomach.

A fine stomach tube is passed through the nose or mouth and into the stomach. Then 150–250 ml of warm, boiled, sterile water (to which a trace of sodium bicarbonate may be added) are introduced through a funnel attached to the tube. The gastric contents are mixed by injecting air through a syringe likewise attached, they are then aspirated into a sterile bottle and cultured.

Laryngeal swab

A laryngeal swab consists of a piece of wire with cotton wool round the end. This is sterilized and kept in a large test tube. The cotton wool is moistened with sterile water or saline just before use, and the swab is placed over the tongue so that the cotton wool is in the pharynx, just above the larynx. When the patient coughs, small flecks of sputum are caught on the cotton wool, these can then be cultured.

The tuberculin test

This test can show that a person has been infected with the tubercle bacillus even though no signs of disease can be found in the lungs or other parts of the body.

Tuberculin is a liquid containing the specific protein which makes up the body of the tubercle bacillus. One preparation is called old tuberculin and is made from a six-week-old culture of tubercle bacilli in glycerol broth. This is evaporated to one-tenth of its volume, sterilized by heat and then filtered. Purified protein derivative (tuberculin PPD) is now used to an increasing extent in place of old tuberculin, since it is constant in composition and potency and (being free from other proteins) does not give non-specific reactions. Tuberculin PPD is prepared from cultures of tubercle bacilli grown in a synthetic medium.

When a person acquires a tuberculous infection, his tissues become hypersensitive to the specific proteins of the bacilli about six weeks later. At this stage, if a small dose of tuberculin is injected into the skin, a specific tissue reaction occurs at the site of the injection, shown by swelling and possibly blistering. This is called a 'positive tuberculin test'. If the tuberculin test is negative, and is again negative two months later, it is certain that the person has not been infected with tuberculosis. A positive reaction means that tuberculosis is a *possible* cause of the person's symptoms.

The usual tuberculin test is the intracutaneous test of Mantoux. In this, 0.1 ml of a 1:1000 dilution of tuberculin is injected intradermally by means of a fine-needled syringe. The test is read after 48 to 72 hours; if the reaction is positive there will be, at the site of the inoculation, an area of swelling or oedema more than 5 mm in diameter. Any surrounding erythema is ignored. If the test is negative, it can be repeated with 0.1 ml of a 1:100 dilution of tuberculin. For a positive reaction with this strength, an area of oedema at least 8 mm in diameter is necessary. Very occasionally, testing may start with a dilution of 1:10 000 tuberculin if the patient is thought to be very sensitive.

A simpler technique for the tuberculin test is to use the Heaf gun (Fig. 5.7). This contains a ring of six needles and, when the handle is pressed, a spring is released, sending these needles through an end plate. A drop of pure tuberculin (PPD) is placed on the skin of the forearm, and the end plate of the gun is then placed over it. The handle of the gun is pressed, and the needles pass through the

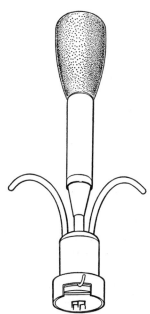

Fig. 5.7 The Heaf gun

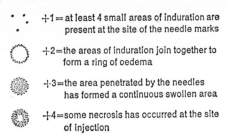

+1 = at least 4 small areas of induration are present at the site of the needle marks

+2 = the areas of induration join together to form a ring of oedema

+3 = the area penetrated by the needles has formed a continuous swollen area

+4 = some necrosis has occurred at the site of injection

Fig. 5.8 The Heaf gun test

solution, taking some into the skin. The performance of this test does not require any skill and the result is best read seven days later, although a positive result is frequently present at 48 hours (Fig. 5.8).

Prevention

Tuberculosis is prevented by eliminating infection and raising the resistance of the community by general and specific measures.

Bovine infection could be eliminated completely by slaughtering all cattle which are shown by the tuberculin test to be infected with the tubercle bacillus, and ensuring that all milk consumed has been pasteurized. However, it will be many years before these objectives are achieved, even in developed countries.

Human tubercle bacilli can be eliminated by finding the human sources of disease, isolating them and rendering them non-infectious. It is also very important to examine the immediate family of newly diagnosed cases of tuberculosis. This is because the circumstances which have made the disease arise in one person are likely to affect other people living under the same conditions and they may well have come into contact with the same source. A tuberculin test is also carried out on contacts and is repeated two months later on those who are negative.

Raising the resistance of the community involves raising the standard of living and providing better housing and working conditions. Education in hygiene, nutrition and the value of fresh air are also important. The resistance of the population can also be raised by *BCG vaccination*. BCG, the bacillus Calmette–Guérin, is a bovine bacillus which has lost a great deal of its virulence by prolonged culture on artificial media. It is given only to people who are tuberculin negative. The vaccination produces a benign primary infection so that the person becomes tuberculin positive. The site of inoculation is usually high up on the arm. After three weeks, a small nodule usually appears on the skin, and some enlargement of the glands of the axilla may occur. In some people, the nodule ulcerates and then heals, leaving a small scar.

Treatment of respiratory tuberculosis

Up to 1950, the basis of the treatment of pulmonary tuberculosis was rest, fresh air and good food. Some doubt has been cast on the value of fresh air, since the results of treatment in Central London have been the same as those in the mountains of Switzerland. Doubts have also been expressed about the value of bed rest in the treatment of tuberculosis. The Medical Research Council Unit in Madras in India found that, provided adequate chemotherapy was given, the patients remaining active at home improved as much as those treated with chemotherapy and bed rest in hospital.

Anybody suspected of having pulmonary tuberculosis should, ideally, be admitted to hospital for a short period. This allows investigations to be carried out and a full bacteriological examination of his sputum to be made. Before specific drugs were available for the treatment of tuberculosis, up to 50 per cent of sputum-positive cases were dead within two years of diagnosis. Nowadays, provided that the organisms are fully sensitive to the main drugs, and that the proper dosage is taken for the full period, almost all patients recover fully.

If admission for investigation is the local policy, segregation but not isolation of these patients is required. They do not need to be confined to bed. The circumstances that makes the admission of patients necessary are:

a. Severe illness
b. Infectious patients
c. Patients, who if left at home, will infect children
d. Those who are unlikely to comply with treatment, either because of their way of life or because of language difficulties

For such patients the nursing care consists of bed rest until the patient's fever has subsided and he is no longer infectious. Admission to a side ward with other patients suffering from pulmonary tuberculosis is preferable to isolation.

Although barrier nursing is not necessary, all crockery and cultery must be boiled for five minutes after use in those hospitals who do not have a central meals service for the wards. The most convenient way to do this is by boiling the utensils from the entire ward;

in this way extraneous organisms are disposed of at the same time. The domestic staff will have to be instructed in the use of the sterilizer and supervision is necessary at intervals to ensure that it really is boiled for five minutes. When the purpose of the procedure has been understood most domestic staff co-operate willingly.

The severely ill patient will need attention to pressure areas and help with personal hygiene and they must be encouraged to move in bed. It is common practice among Asians in particular to sit cross-legged on their beds for long periods: this puts pressure on their calf muscles and has been known to give rise to deep vein thrombosis and pulmonary embolus. The habit should be discouraged. Generally the patient is allowed up to wash and toilet – remaining in bed for the rest of the time until the temperature has subsided, the sputum is negative to direct smear examination and the X-ray appearances of the lesion are showing improvement. Linen should be simply put in a labelled bag and sent to the laundry to be washed in the normal way. Paper handkerchiefs are used, collected in a paper bag and burnt daily. Disposable sputum cartons with screw-on lids are provided, instruction should be given to keep the lid screwed on when not in use – this avoids unnecessary contamination if knocked over. They are collected daily and are incinerated with the handkerchiefs. Patients who have difficulty in removing and replacing the lids of these cartons may be given stainless steel sputum mugs in the bottom of which is placed some antiseptic.

The steel mugs should be collected daily on a steel tray with high sides. They should be autoclaved at a pressure of 12–15 lbs per square inch for fifteen minutes. The special autoclave then empties the sputum down the drain.

If a patient with tuberculosis is treated at home he should be provided with a sputum flask which he can carry in his pocket. After last using the flask at night he should add 50 ml of bleach and leave it for an hour after which the liquid can be emptied down the lavatory. The flask should then be washed. If the outside has been contaminated the flask should be boiled after the top has been removed.

The diet should be high in protein to help build up broken down tissue. Many of our patients with tuberculosis in this country today are of Asian origin adhering to a strict vegetarian diet. These diets are low in protein and iron so we have an anaemic patient who finds it aesthetically unacceptable on religious grounds or through custom to eat the diet provided and recommended. Some vegetarians will eat fish and eggs, others can sometimes be persuaded to do so. There is a strong family bond of respect to elders and those in authority in the extended family of Asian immigrants and the nurse who seeks the co-operation of the husband, father or mother-in-law, as is appropriate, is most likely to meet with success in her efforts. It may be necessary to enlist the aid of an interpreter, particularly if the mother-in-law is to be approached: if so, make certain that the interpreter speaks the same language. Hospital vegetarian diets are likely to become monotonous and relatives may be encouraged to bring a meal from time to time – this will be far more acceptable to the patient than anything else.

It must be clearly understood that the drug regime is the key to recovery and the nurse has a duty to imbue a respect for the medications which will endure for the 9–15 months of the treatment. This can be done by giving them at the same time each day and simply insisting that they are taken under supervision.

Gastro-intestinal disturbance, skin rash, a rise in temperature or disturbance of vision should be regarded as possible drug reactions and reported to the medical staff forthwith.

These problems, if they do occur, present commonly during the first twenty-one days of treatment, hence the advantage of having the patient in hospital.

Financial hardship is an obstacle to recovery and hospitalisation may well affect the family income. The patient may not wish to discuss these matters with the ward staff, on the other hand anxiety can lead to a stress situation giving rise to misunderstandings. The astute nurse will quickly introduce the medical social worker who will be able to arrange for supplementary benefit, if appropriate. There are arrangements that can be made with employers and Building Societies which can put the patient's mind at rest. If there is a language difficulty there is a very real need for this kind of help.

Occupational therapy is invariably arranged by the patient himself in the form of books, games study, puzzles etc. Television provides contact with the world outside the ward but it should be provided with earphones so that the noise is not inflicted on unwilling ears.

Drug treatment consists of the oral administration of the three main drugs–Rifampicin, (600 mg daily for those over 40 Kg body weight and 450 mg daily for those under this weight) Ethambutol, 15–17 mg per Kg body weight) and Isoniazid (5 mg per Kg body weight). These drugs are given once daily, Rifampicin on an empty stomach before breakfast and the other two after breakfast.

Because of past errors in treatment, drug resistance is prevalent in many parts of the world and so all newly diagnosed cases of tuberculosis are treated with these drugs until the examination of cultures has shown that the organism is sensitive to all of them. Treatment is then continued with a combination of two drugs. Usually this consists of Rifampicin and Isoniazid which is the most powerful combination known. Since the administration of one drug alone leads to the development of resistance, the two drugs are usually given combined either as Rimactazid or Rifinah. The chemotherapy is continued for nine months and is so effective that, provided the patient has been assiduous in taking them, relapse is almost unknown. Tubercle bacilli are usually eliminated from the sputum within a few weeks, but in an occasional case sputum conversion may be delayed.

Drug reactions are few. Rifampicin causes the urine to be orange-red in colour and discolouration of the sputum, tears and sweat with slight staining of the clothes. Rifampicin should not be used in the presence of jaundice or pregnancy and since the drug inactivates the contraceptive pill any woman taking this form of contraception should have the dosage doubled. Occasionally gastrointestinal upset occurs, drug rashes and purpura. A transient disturbance of liver function occurs. If this persists the drug must be discontinued.

Side effects to Isoniazid are very uncommon. Skin rashes and dimness of vision have occurred. The most serious side effect is peripheral neuritis producing muscular weakness and a burning sensation in the limbs. This can be prevented and cured by giving Vitamin B_6 (Pyridoxin) 10 mg daily.

The main side effect of Ethambutol is visual impairment due to optic neuritis and is related to the dosage and duration of treatment.

Any change in vision must be reported immediately and the drug stopped. Recovery usually occurs in weeks or months. Occasionally gynaecomastia occurs.

When the patient is resistant to two of the three drugs, then others must be used. These are frequently more toxic and less effective in overcoming the tuberculosis and are sometimes referred to as 'salvage' drugs. When sputum conversion is delayed with the standard treatment, one or more of these might be added to the regime. The drugs include Streptomycin, Ethionamide, Pyrazinamide, Viomycin and Cycloserine.

Before the discovery of adequate chemotherapy for the treatment of tuberculosis, deliberate collapse of the damaged lung was a frequent mode of treatment (Fig. 5.9). Collapse therapy is not now used, but the nurse may come across patients who have had this

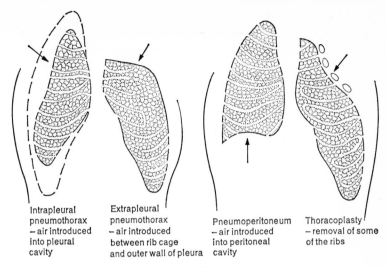

Intrapleural pneumothorax – air introduced into pleural cavity

Extrapleural pneumothorax – air introduced between rib cage and outer wall of pleura

Pneumoperitoneum – air introduced into peritoneal cavity

Thoracoplasty – removal of some of the ribs

Fig. 5.9 Artificially induced collapse of the lung

treatment in the past. A similar form of treatment was a permanent collapse of the lung produced by a *thoracoplasty* (see also Fig. 7.2, p. 132). In this operation, parts of the upper eight ribs were removed so that the side of the chest wall fell in and compressed the underlying lung. Surgical removal of part of a lung which has been damaged by tuberculosis is still occasionally carried out.

After discharge from hospital, the patient continues to attend the out-patient department for follow-up. A person diagnosed as having tuberculosis is reported to the District Community Physician so that arrangements can be made for the examination of contacts.

Bronchiectasis

This is a condition in which the smaller bronchi of the lungs become permanently dilated, either in a regular fashion (*tubular bronchiectasis*) or in an irregular fashion (*saccular bronchiectasis*). The disease may sometimes be generalized throughout the lungs, either as a complication of chronic bronchitis or due to a congenital defect of the bronchi. However it is far more frequently localized in one or two lobes of the lungs, usually at the bases.

Permanent dilatation of the bronchial tubes occurs only when prolonged obstruction is complicated by infection. When part of the lung collapses, the bronchi and the other parts of the lung expand to help fill the space. Normally, when the collapsed lobe re-expands, the bronchi return to their original size. However, if infection is present in the bronchial wall, this destroys its smooth muscle and elastic tissue. The epithelium which lines the bronchi loses its cilia, and the entire bronchial wall may be replaced by fibrous tissue with the formation of little sacs. Newly formed fibrous tissue usually contracts with time, and this contraction causes distortion of the bronchi. Because the cilia have been lost and the bronchi have become rigid, secretions are not removed and this stagnation leads to further lung damage. The posterior parts of the lower lobes are most commonly involved, since this is where most of the secretions in the bronchial tree will settle during sleep. The anterior segments are sometimes involved in children who sleep face down.

Before the introduction of antibiotics and immunization programmes, bronchiectasis commonly followed whooping cough, measles and influenza. Today, bronchopneumonia is the most likely preceding cause. Aspiration of a foreign body, particularly in children and, in adults, obstruction from a bronchial carcinoma, frequently lead to the development of bronchiectasis, as can primary tuberculosis. When the disease results from bronchial obstruction due to thick secretions in chronic bronchitis and bronchial asthma, it is patchy in distribution and scattered throughout both lungs.

The clinical features of bronchiectasis vary, depending more on the amount of infection in the affected bronchi than on the amount of lung damage. Patients fall into three groups:

a. The bronchiectasis may show no symptoms for many years. Infection then occurs and extensive involvement of the lungs is found. In spite of this, further symptoms may not occur again for many years.

b. Classical bronchiectasis – there is usually a history here of recurrent episodes of cough, often since childhood, with the production of a considerable amount of purulent sputum (sometimes containing blood). In winter, the condition becomes worse, with increased cough and sputum after each cold. If the lower lobe of only one lung is involved, the patient will frequently complain he is wakened at night with the coughing up of foul, thick, green sputum whenever he turns over on to the side of the healthy lung. Even in quiet periods, the patient finds that talking has to be interrupted in order to cough. There is a great deal of sputum in the mornings, and the patient may vomit with his bouts of coughing, or even faint. Some patients bring up each day as much as half a litre of frothy smelling sputum which usually separates into three layers in the sputum mug. The bottom layer consists of pus cell, plugs of mucus and organisms, the middle layer is a watery solution, and the top layer is froth.

c. The dry type of bronchiectasis (*bronchiectasis sicca*) may have haemoptysis as the sole symptom. The patient may cough up as much as 250 to 500 ml of pure blood. This type of bronchiectasis is frequently restricted to the upper lobes. Shortness of breath may be a prominent symptom in older patients when the disease is diffuse, and chronic bronchitis frequently supervenes at this stage.

In classical bronchiectasis the patient appears chronically ill. There is often marked clubbing of the fingers (Fig. 5.10) and toes, tenderness over the nasal sinuses due to infection, and a mild anaemia. In an established case, a chest X-ray may not show any abnormality, but in others linear shadows occur from the root of the lung to the periphery. Triangular shadows of lobar collapse may be seen at either lung base, especially in children. The extent of the disease can be determined by *bronchography* – a procedure in which the bronchial tree is outlined on an X-ray film using an aqueous iodine preparation called Dionosil.

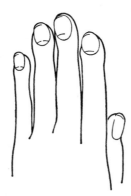

Fig. 5.10 Clubbing of the fingers in bronchiectasis

Bronchography

An X-ray film of a normal lung shows only a fine pattern produced mainly by the blood vessels. The larger bronchial tubes can be shown up by introducing an aqueous iodine solution through which X-rays cannot pass, so that a shadow appears on the film. The bronchi must first be cleared of secretions by placing the patient in different positions (see p. 94) and getting him to cough up all the secretions he can. When the sputum is copious, postural coughing must be carried out for several days if an adequate bronchogram is to be obtained.

No premedication is usually necessary but, in nervous patients diazepam (10 mg) may be given beforehand. A 100 mg benzocaine lozenge is sucked until it dissolves, and the throat is sprayed with a 1 per cent solution of benzocaine. After a short wait, a sterilized rubber tube is passed through one nostril, through the pharynx and into the trachea. The aqueous iodine solution is then injected through this rubber tube into the bronchi, using a 50 ml syringe. The patient is placed in such a position that the solution runs into the desired part of the lung and an X-ray film is then taken (Fig. 5.11). Where there is difficulty in passing a tube through the nose into the trachea (e.g., because the nasal septum is deformed) a needle is inserted directly into the trachea through its anterior wall.

After the bronchogram has been performed the patient is again given postural drainage for two to three hours to remove as much of the iodine solution from the lung as possible. The rest is completely absorbed in two to three days.

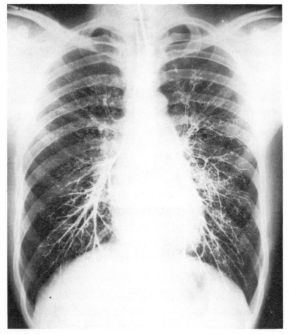

Fig. 5.11A A normal bronchogram

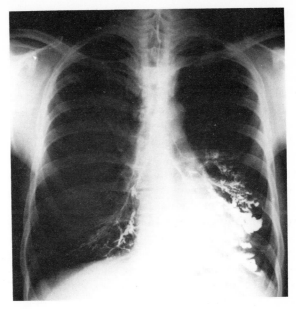

Fig. 5.11B A bronchogram showing bronchiectasis

An X-ray of the nasal sinuses often shows infection. The sinuses may have been infected first (with aspiration of the resulting pus into the lung causing the bronchiectasis), or they may have been infected from the lung.

The course of the disease is extremely variable. In some patients the life span is not affected. In others brain abscess, amyloid disease, haemorrhage or failure of the right side of the heart may occur.

Treatment

Hospitalisation is not necessary unless bronchoscopic investigation is indicated or acute pulmonary infection develops. The opportunity can be taken to re-educate the patient and the family about postural drainage, breathing exercises, medications and the importance of a well balanced diet with adequate fluid content to enable viscous sputum to be drained and expectorated.

Where the disease is not too extensive and where there is no coincident asthma or bronchitis, removal of the damaged part of the lung may be the best treatment. This is especially so in cases of bronchiectasis sicca, when recurrent haemoptyses are quite frightening to the patient.

In most cases the patient is treated medically rather than surgically. This treatment consists of the use of postural drainage (see Fig. 4.11, p. 72) and the administration of antibiotics. The patient is taught the position in which the secretions will drain from the bronchiectatic area toward the main bronchus and trachea. The lower lobe is affected in the great majority of patients, and postural drainage for this lobe is achieved by leaning face downwards over the side of the bed with the hands on the floor. Postural drainage of the right middle lobe or left lingular process is achieved by placing the patient on his back with the foot of the bed raised. With upper lobe bronchiectasis, drainage will take place if the patient is sitting up and leaning towards the unaffected side. The appropriate position must be adopted for at least ten minutes twice a day and during this time forcible coughing should be continued until no more sputum is brought up. Drainage of the secretions can often be improved by placing one hand on the chest over the affected lobe and hitting this hand with the clenched fist of the other hand. A physiotherapist should carry out this procedure at first, but the nurse or patient's relatives can continue it. During periods of acute infection, antibiotic therapy is guided by the results of sputum cultures. In patients who suffer repeated episodes of acute infection, or whose sputum is persistently purulent, small doses of antibiotics may be given continuously through the winter months. Periodic culture of the sputum should be obtained during such therapy to ensure that resistant organisms have not emerged.

Sarcoidosis

Sarcoidosis is a disease whose cause is not known. Fleshy (*granulomatous*), inflammatory lesions appear in many organs of the body, but especially in the lungs. The appearance of sarcoid tissue under the microscope is very similar to tuberculosis. However, the centre of the lesion does not become caseous (cheesy) in appearance as in tuberculosis. Many doctors think that sarcoidosis is an atypical form of tuberculosis, but others do not. The disease is most common among young people, particularly women.

The symptoms of sarcoidosis are mild. The presenting feature may be *erythema nodosum*, a condition in which bluish-red lumps appear on the skin, usually on the front of the legs. Other symptoms include mild fever, loss of weight, and lack of energy. A cough is rare. If the parotid glands are involved, the facial nerve may be paralysed, producing a facial palsy. Involvement of the eye gives rise to iritis.

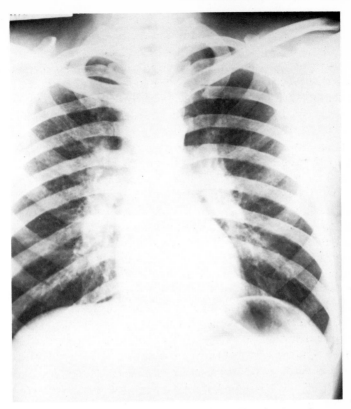

Fig. 5.12 An X-ray showing enlargement of the hilar glands at the root of the lung in a case of sarcoidosis

The disease is most frequently diagnosed by a routine chest X-ray. The hilar glands at the root of the lung are usually enlarged (Fig. 5.12). In other patients, pulmonary infiltration is present, with fine or coarse scattered nodular opacities and sometimes scattered patches (Fig. 5.13). In most cases the radiological changes slowly settle over a period of years but, in a minority, pulmonary fibrosis occurs.

Characteristically, the tuberculin test is negative. If BCG vaccination (see p. 84) is given, the tuberculin test fails to become positive afterwards. A skin test called the *Kveim test* is of some value in diagnosis. This consists of the injection of extract of sarcoid tissue into the skin of the forearm. At the site of injection a small nodule develops during the next four to six weeks and a biopsy of this nodule shows the microscopic appearance of sarcoidosis.

The main method of diagnosing sarcoidosis is by finding the histological changes typical of the process in some of the tissues in the

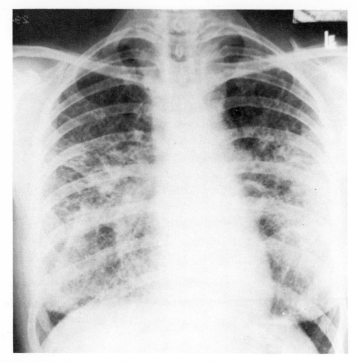

Fig. 5.13 An X-ray showing pulmonary infiltration in case of sarcoidosis

body. Commonly the surgeon carries out a *scalene node biopsy*. This involves removing one of the lymph glands behind the scalene muscle in the neck for histological examination. Alternatively a blind lung biopsy can be performed using the fibre-optic flexible bronchoscope. This is passed in the usual way into the trachea and then under control of the x-ray screen the bronchoscope is pushed down one of the smaller bronchi until it will not pass any further. Screening ensures that the tip of the bronchoscope is not close to the visceral pleura and a biopsy of lung tissue is then taken. Complications are small haemoptyses and the development of a pneumothorax.

Treatment

In most cases all that is necessary is a short rest in bed until the general symptoms have cleared. In a few cases, steroid treatment is used. The one danger in pulmonary sarcoidosis is the development of fibrosis, as this may cause considerable dyspnoea after a number of years.

The nursing care is minimal, consisting of a simple explanation of each investigation as it is done and encouragement to persevere with bed rest, which is frequently irksome to the patient who does not feel ill and resenting the interruption in his life.

Pneumoconiosis

The pneumoconioses are a group of diseases caused by the inhalation of dust into the lungs. The most common is *coal-workers' pneumoconiosis*, which is frequently encountered in mining communities. It occurs in two forms, *simple pneumoconiosis* (which is fairly mild) and *progressive massive fibrosis* (which causes severe dyspnoea and cough, accompanied by black-stained sputum). Disablement and death may follow. Prevention of the disease is difficult, and there is no specific treatment.

Other types of pneumoconiosis include *silicosis* (which also occurs in coal miners, and in the granite and sandstone industries), *asbestosis* (which occurs after prolonged exposure to asbestos, i.e. magnesium silicate dust) and *byssinosis* (which is due to inhalation of cotton dust). The features of all these conditions are broadly similar to those of coal-workers' pneumoconiosis. These diseases are uncommon except in industrial areas where dusts of the types mentioned are generated.

Pulmonary fibrosis causes ventilatory and diffusion dysfunction resulting from rigid lung tissue and may therefore be regarded as a restrictive pulmonary disease. The nursing care however is similar to that of obstructive airways disease as described on page 53.

Six
Tumours of the chest

Lung cancer

Over the last thirty years mortality rates for most of the important sites of cancer have either shown little variation or have decreased. Thus, the incidence of cancer of the breast is approximately the same as it was in the 1930s (Fig. 6.1).

The incidene of cancer of the lung, however, has risen steadily, and it is now one of the most common lung diseases. All patients of middle or advanced years with chest symptoms must be suspected

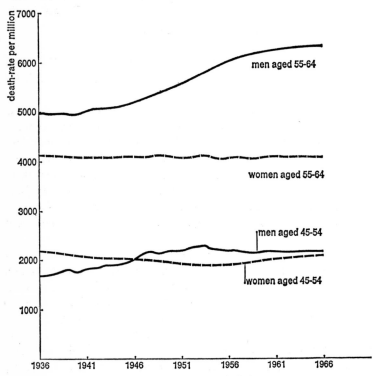

Fig. 6.1 Death-rate per million for cancer of all sites

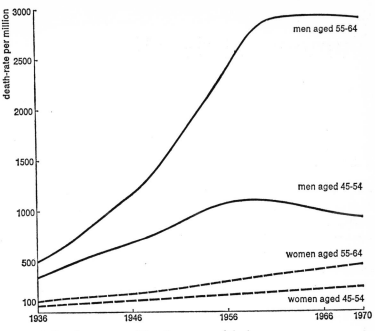

Fig. 6.2 Death-rate per million for cancer of the lung

of having a bronchial carcinoma until proved otherwise. However, cancer of the lung is not unknown even in people in their thirties or, very rarely, in their twenties.

A significant feature of the statistics is the difference between the rates for men and for women. The lung is now the most common site for cancer in men, and this disease is responsible for 35 per cent of all cancer deaths in England and Wales. Recently the rate, especially for middle-aged men, seems to be levelling off and there has been a slight decrease for men aged forty-five to fifty-four. Among women, lung cancer accounts for only 7 per cent of all cancer deaths but, although the rate is low compared with men, it is rising sharply (Fig. 6.2).

The cause of lung cancer (or indeed of most cancers) is not yet fully understood, but the causal relationship with smoking is well established. While many other factors may have had a bearing on the differences noted between mortality rates from lung cancer in men and women, the only factor that has altered radically in recent years is the consumption of tobacco (Fig. 6.3). Investigations have shown that in those who smoke twenty cigarettes per day or more, 10 per cent will eventually die of a bronchial carcinoma. The rising incidence among women appears to be related to the increasing

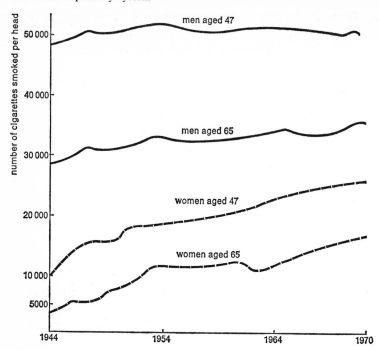

Fig. 6.3 Number of cigarettes smoked per head over the previous ten years

number who now smoke cigarettes. Opinions differ as to whether pipe and cigar tobacco is also carcinogenic, but any risk would appear to be very much less than that associated with cigarettes.

Atmospheric pollution in towns may also be a factor in producing bronchial carcinoma. Among non-smokers, the incidence of lung cancer is higher in industrial areas than in rural areas. Among cigarette smokers, there is virtually no difference in lung cancer incidence between city and country dwellers.

No evidence has been found that diesel fumes are responsible for lung cancer. The disease does, however, occur in those who work in certain industries, notably the mining of radioactive materials, the manufacture of chromates and coal gas, and the processing of arsenic and asbestos.

Types of tumour

Three types of bronchial carcinoma are described, according to the cell type which is found on examination under the microscope:

a. Squamous. This is slow growing and is the most common type. Some of these tumours which grow more quickly may be reported by the pathologist as being undifferentiated carcinomas.

b. Oat Cell. These tumours are also common. They have a very characteristic appearance under the microscope. They grow quickly and give rise to secondary cancers in other organs of the body early in the disease. They are therefore less likely to be operable than the squamous type. This type of tumour also often has the peculiar power of producing chemicals which resemble the hormones secreted by various endocrine glands, so that diseases other than lung cancer may be mimicked.

c. Adenocarcinoma. This type of tumour is uncommon. It has cells which are columnar in shape and, unlike the other two types, does

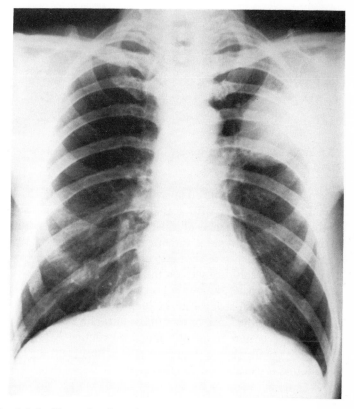

Fig. 6.4 An X-ray showing a lung cancer as a peripheral shadow in the lung

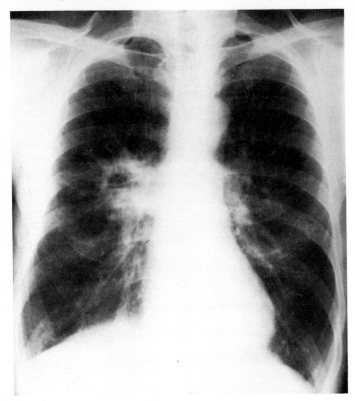

Fig. 6.5 An X-ray showing peripheral cancer breaking down in the centre to form a cavity

not seem to have any connection with cigarette smoking. It arises frequently in association with scars in the lung. These scars are often the result of small areas of inflammation which occur during a chest infection. This type of tumour is more frequent in women and has a great tendency to seed into other parts of the lung so that multiple round nodules are seen on the chest X-ray.

Whatever the type of tumour, a lung cancer is seen radiologically as either a peripheral shadow in the lung (Figs. 6.4 and 6.5) or as an enlargement of the *hilum* or root of the lung (Fig. 6.6).

Lung cancer is now frequently found on routine X-rays of the chest. There are usually no symptoms at this stage, and the type of tumour found is usually peripheral in type.

Symptoms

The most common symptom of lung cancer is the presence of a

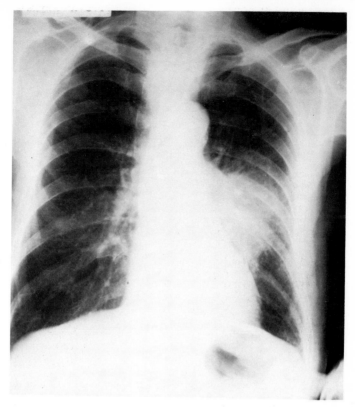

Fig. 6.6 An X-ray showing enlargement of the left hilum

chest infection which fails to clear up within two or three weeks. Other possible symptoms include haemoptysis (see p. 23), blood-spitting, pain, shortness of breath, general ill-health, weight loss and muscle wasting.

Since both chronic bronchitis and bronchial carcinoma may arise from cigarette smoking, the two are frequently found together. In such cases the chronic bronchitic may complain that his cough has changed its character and is now more persistent or that his sputum is now heavily blood-stained.

The development of pneumonia may also be a symptom of lung cancer. Since the hilar type of growth arises in the wall of one of the larger bronchi and usually grows round the wall, narrowing of the bronchus occurs. This can result in the collapse of the part of the lung supplied by that bronchus (Fig. 6.7). Infection of this collapsed lung then occurs, resulting in pneumonia. This infection will

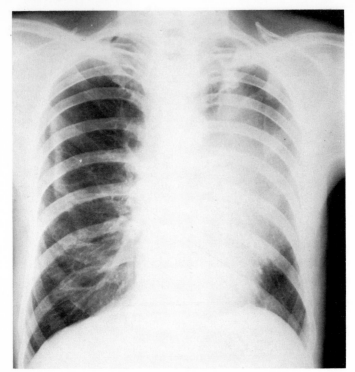

Fig. 6.7 An X-ray showing collapse of the left upper lobe of the lung due to cancer

clear satisfactorily with antibiotics, but may well recur. Patients over forty, even after they appear to have recovered from pneumonia, should always have a chest X-ray taken to ensure that no underlying bronchial carcinoma is present. The same routine should apply to cases of lung abscess, which are frequently secondary to the obstruction of a bronchus by a carcinoma.

A bout of pneumonia which is secondary to a bronchial carcinoma may be followed by the appearance of a pleural effusion. This effusion usually clears with aspiration and the treatment of the pneumonia with the appropriate antibiotics. A pleural effusion may also develop if a tumour invades the pleura, or if cancer blocks the lymph glands which drain the lung (Fig. 6.8).

A bronchial carcinoma can occur with no respiratory symptoms. Sometimes the tumour presents as an endocrine disorder. A bronchial carcinoma, especially the oat cell variety, can produce chemicals which the body cannot differentiate from hormones produced by the pituitary gland. These changes include increased secretion of

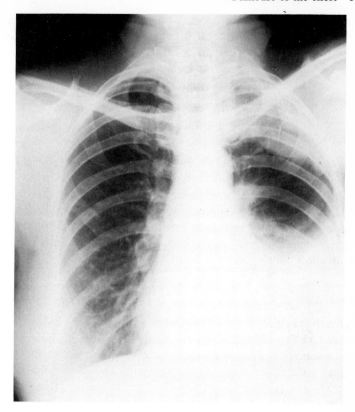

Fig. 6.8 An X-ray showing a large right pleural effusion due to cancer

the cortex of the supra renal gland (Cushing's Syndrome), hyper-thyroidism, hyper para-thyroidism, hypoglycaemia and enlarge-ment of the breasts (gynaecomastia). Hoarseness can occur if a vo-cal cord is paralysed. This is because the recurrent laryngeal nerve which supplies the larynx passes through the chest and may be compressed by a tumour growing there.

A carcinoma which arises in the apex of the lung is called a *Pancoast tumour*. It frequently invades the sympathetic nerves, causing constriction of the pupil of the eye on the same side, drooping of the upper eyelid and sinking in of the eyeball. This group of findings is known as *Horner's syndrome*. It is frequently associated with pain in the shoulder due to involvement of the brachial plexus.

Secondary spread to the glands in the mediastinum can cause pressure on the oesophagus and hence difficulty in swallowing (*dysphagia*). Superior vena caval obstruction can also occur so that the veins of the head, neck and upper limbs become distended. The patient usually complains that his neck is getting bigger and his collars do not fit. The face appears swollen and blue. Some patients have symptoms of a brain tumour, since many brain growths are secondary to a lung cancer. In some patients skin nodules from metastases are first noticed.

Investigations

Most patients are admitted for investigation of a possible lung cancer because of an abnormal chest X-ray, although in some it may be because of a persistent unexplained cough or because they have brought up some blood-stained sputum and are heavy smokers.

All patients should have their temperature, pulse and respiration rate recorded and their urine tested. Sputum is sent to the laboratory to check for the presence of malignant cells.

Bronchoscopy

This is the most common routine investigation. A *bronchoscope* consists of a hollow tube about 35 cm long with a smaller illuminating tube alongside it (Fig. 6.9). There are several holes at the side through which the patient is able to breathe even if the end of the bronchoscope is obstructed. Bronchoscopy is usually, though not always, carried out under a general anaesthetic.

An explanation of the procedure should be given to the patient and his relative and a consent form signed. No food or drink is given for four hours prior to the investigation. The bladder is emptied and he is dressed in an operation gown and pyjama trou-

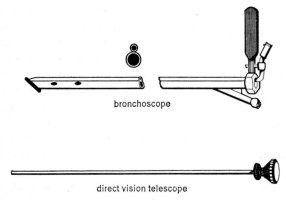

bronchoscope

direct vision telescope

Fig. 6.9 A bronchoscope

sers and a premedication is given. The screens are pulled round the bed and he is advised to relax and try to sleep. Just before the anaesthetic is given, the patient should gargle with 15 ml of 4 per cent xylocaine. This anaesthetizes the pharynx and makes it less likely that he will cough.

The general anaesthetic used is frequently nitrous oxide and oxygen given through a mask and combined with pentothal intravenously. A muscle relaxant is usually given; this may make the patient's muscles ache next day, so he should be warned that this might occur.

The patient is placed on his back on the operating table. His head is lowered so that the mouth, pharynx and trachea are in a straight line, and the bronchoscope is inserted into the pharynx. Both sides of the bronchial tree are examined by direct vision and with the telescope. Secretions in the bronchial tree are removed by means of a sucker and, if any abnormal area is seen, a small piece of tissue is removed with biopsy forceps so that it can be examined under the microscope. Both these types of specimen are placed in small bottles containing formol saline, obtained from the pathological laboratory. They must be labelled with the patient's name and hospital number by the attending nurse *as soon as they have been taken* so that no mistake in identity can be made. Mistakes in labelling biopsy specimens are common and unfortunate consequences can follow.

Complications during the operation are rare, although spasm of the larynx and oedema of the glottis can occur. Haemorrhage is uncommon unless a biopsy has been taken. These complications are usually dealt with by the surgeon and anaesthetist, but the nurse must be prepared to produce a resuscitation tray and apparatus for giving an intravenous drip of blood, plasma or saline.

In the recovery room, the patient must be observed closely, since he may stop breathing and need artificial respiration and oxygen, or may cough up a large amount of blood. In either eventuality, the doctor must be summoned immediately. On returning to the ward, the patient is laid in the lateral position, so that his tongue does not fall back into the throat, and he is kept under observation until he recovers from the anaesthetic. He must not be given anything to eat or drink for three hours afterwards, since the throat is still anaesthetized and food may be aspirated into the trachea and lungs. He should be reassured that it is customary to cough up some blood-stained sputum after a biopsy has been taken.

Bronchoscopy aids diagnosis where the tumour is in one of the major bronchi, but this is the only part of the bronchial tree which can be visualized. Even when a right-angled telescope is used, only the opening of the upper lobe bronchus can be seen. The examination is then often supplemented by using a flexible fibreoptic bronchoscope.

Light can be carried along a minute glass fibre so that it only appears at the end as a result of total internal reflection. This phenomenon is used in those table decorations which look like a sunburst where different coloured lights come out of the ends of the individual fibres but the fibres themselves appear to be colourless.

In a fibre-endoscope, such as a bronchoscope, thousands of such very fine glass fibres are bound together in a flexible bundle so that the light reflected by an object is conducted along the fibre bundle. This object can then be viewed by an observer using an eyepiece at the other end of the bundle.

The proximal end of the bronchoscope, which is held in the hand, contains an eyepiece for viewing, a light source, controls to move the tip of the other end, valves to control suction and an opening through which biopsy forceps can be introduced. The flexible shaft resembles a thin black snake and can be up to a metre in length. The distal tip can be bent back upon itself in all four directions, making entry into small bronchi easy.

This instrument can be used to supplement examination with the ordinary bronchoscope by passing the flexible tube along the rigid bronchoscope and examining further any bronchus which looks suspicious.

Sometimes the instrument is used alone. This procedure can be carried out with the patient propped up in bed. Valium 5 mg is given orally half an hour before. The flexible bronchoscope is then inserted through which of the nasal passages appears to be the larger and passed down through the pharynx. When the vocal cords are seen in the eyepiece lignocaine is sprayed on them and the tube is then passed between the cords and the different bronchi visualised in turn. Disturbance to the patient is slight and there is no special post operative care. Unfortunately the biopsy specimens obtained through the fibreoptic bronchoscope are minute and the pathologist sometimes has difficulty in interpreting the microscope slides made from the specimens obtained.

When the cancer is much further out in the peripheral part of the lung, bronchoscopy is useless unless the glands in the root of the lung have become enlarged by secondary deposits. Occasionally for these peripheral tumours needle biopsy is done through the chest wall under X-ray screening control.

Tomography

With peripheral tumours, tomography (or 'layer X-rays') can be helpful in obtaining a clear X-ray picture of a very small area of lung.

Tomography is a special technique in which the X-ray film and X-ray tube are connected together by a long metal rod, pivoted near the middle (Fig. 6.10). As the X-ray tube is pushed from the patient's head to his feet in an arc, the film travels from his feet to his head. During this process, only a small layer of the lung about 1 cm thick is in focus on the plate at a time, and so a picture appears of that layer of the lung only. By altering the position of the pivot, different layers of the lung are brought into focus.

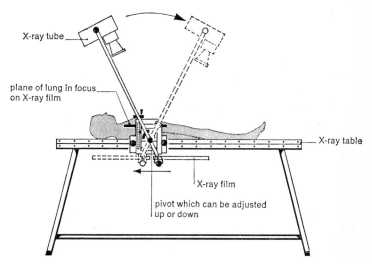

Fig. 6.10 The arrangements for lung tomography

Pleural biopsy

If a pleural effusion is present, a pleural biopsy may show malignant infiltration of the pleura. The pleural biopsy needle is a wide-bore needle with a side opening. Down the centre there is another tube with a sharp cutting end (Fig. 6.11).

The patient sits in an upright position and leans forward over a bed-trolley with his arms resting on a pillow. The skin and the underlying tissues are infiltrated with a local anaesthetic (2 ml of 1 per cent xylocaine) using a syringe and needle. A small incision is

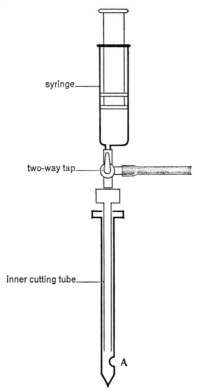

Fig. 6.11 Pleural biopsy needle

then made in the skin with a scalpel, and the pleural biopsy needle (connected to a 10 ml syringe via a two-way tap) is pushed through the chest wall into the fluid. When the plunger of the syringe is withdrawn, fluid is drawn into the barrel. The tap is then turned so that, when the plunger of the syringe is pushed inwards, the fluid passes through the tap and down the rubber tubing into a suitable receptacle (Fig. 6.12). Some of the fluid can be placed in a sterile bottle and sent to the laboratory for examination for the presence of cells – both normal and malignant – and for bacteria.

During the operation the nurse must keep the patient in the correct position and instruct him to try not to cough – since sudden expansion of the lung may result in the needle penetrating the lung. She must also observe the patient's pulse, colour and respiration. If fluid is removed too quickly, the underlying lung (which has been compressed by the fluid) expands quickly, throwing a sudden strain on the pulmonary circulation, and making the patient distressed

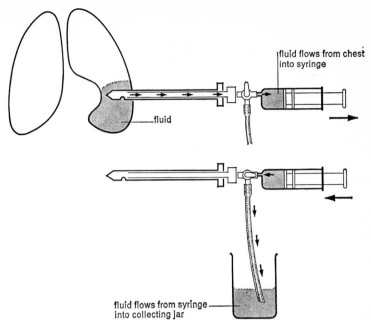

Fig. 6.12 The use of the two-way tap in chest aspiration

and breathless. The fluid is removed until a maximum of 500 ml has been extracted. If more fluid than this is present the procedure must be repeated on another day.

When the aspiration of the chest has been completed, the pleural biopsy needle is withdrawn until the side opening A (Fig. 6.11) catches in the chest wall. The inner tube is then pushed down the inside of the needle so as to cut off a small piece of pleura. This is placed in a bottle containing formol saline for subsequent examination in the laboratory under the microscope. The bottle must be labelled immediately.

After aspiration the nurse must make the patient comfortable, instruct him not to get out of bed by himself for four hours and record the amount of fluid removed. If the liquid is infected, the doctor will give instructions that it must be disinfected before disposal.

Treatment of lung cancer

The overall outlook for any case of bronchial carcinoma is extremely poor, which is why cigarette smoking is so dangerous. At present the main treatment with any chance of success is surgical removal of the growth and the associated part of the lung, together with the lymph glands draining it. Of one hundred newly-diagnosed cases of lung cancer, twenty-five have their growth removed, but only six of these patients will be alive five years after operation. Thus, cure of lung cancer is rare.

The operation of choice, if possible, is removal of one lobe (*lobectomy*). Removal of an entire lung (*pneumonectomy*) may make an older patient a respiratory cripple.

The operation

Admission to the surgical ward takes place several days before the elected date of operation. This enables the patient and the caring team to get to know each other. The blood group and haemoglobin will be determined. If he is anaemic a blood transfusion will be given to bring his haemoglobin level up to normal. The physiotherapist teaches breathing exercises and instructs him how to cough easily, using his diaphragm only. This is because movement of the chest will be painful after operation. The medical staff will interview the next of kin. The anaesthetist will visit the patient and order a suitable pre-medication. On the evening before the operation the nurse must check:

a. That the patient has signed the consent form
b. That an adequate supply of blood of the right group is available
c. That the operation site is shaved
d. That the patient has had a bath
e. That a night sedative has been written up by the doctor to ensure that the patient has a good night's sleep

On the day of operation the nurse must check:

a. Foods and fluids are stopped from midnight
b. Urine has been tested for abnormalities
c. An early morning bath is given
d. The patient is dressed in operation gown and stockings
e. Dentures and any other artifical appliances are removed
f. The patient's notes and identity badge are checked against each other
g. A check is made that the doctor has marked the patient's name and site of operation on the arm bracelet or skin
h. The premedication is given as written on the treatment sheet.
i. The patient is left in a quiet area so that he can sleep as the premedication takes effect

j. A nurse accompanies the patient to the operating theatre, making sure that she has the correct notes and X-rays

The operation is carried out with the patient lying on his side. The surgeon usually opens the thoracic cavity by removing part of the fifth rib through an incision which extends from near the spine to the lateral side of the chest. The affected lobe (or whole lung) is removed by dividing and tying the pulmonary arteries and veins and oversewing the bronchial stump. Since a good deal of blood is lost during the operation a transfusion is always set up (the patient is returned to the ward with this still running). While still unconscious the patient is laid on his back with his head to one side.

Postoperative care of a patient following lobectomy or segmented resection

The routine observation should be taken systematically by the nurse caring for the patient during that tour of duty. It is the store of information that enables her to plan appropriate care and it needs to be related to the base line that was observed prior to operation before she can know what is within normal limits for that particular situation. The following must be observed:

1. The airway is patent
2. Level of consciousness
3. Colour and condition of skin
4. Pulse rate, rhythm and volume
5. Blood pressure
6. The wound is checked to ensure there is no oozing of blood from the suture line
7. The intravenous line is functioning satisfactorily
8. The intercostal tubes are patent

There are always two intercostal tubes in situ after lobectomy or segmental resection and the successful management of these tubes is of prime importance. They are attached to two underwater seal bottles which form an air lock, allowing air and fluid to escape but not allowing air or infection to enter (Fig. 6.13). It must be noted that the tube attached to the patient is connected to the long glass tube which has the end in the sterile water, 1 cm above the bottom of the bottle. The tubes can be seen to be patent when the water in the long glass tube in the bottle oscillates with respiration. This occurs because the end of the tube is in the space between the chest wall and the lung and this space changes in size with respiration. The patient may also be asked to cough. If there is an air leak a

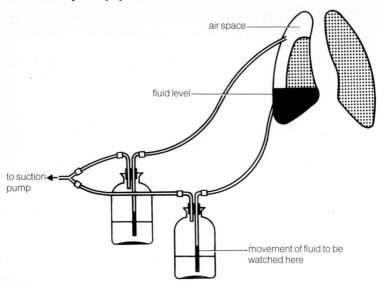

air space

fluid level

to suction
pump

movement of fluid to be
watched here

Fig. 6.13 Underwater drain. Suction from both bottles can be achieved
with one suction pump only and the use of the Y connection.

bubble will escape, again showing the tube to be patent and, of
course, if fluid is draining the tube is not blocked. Obstruction
occurs when fibrin builds up on the wall of the tube and it can be
broken down and removed by 'milking', a process which may be
described as pinching the tube and steadying it with the left hand
whilst drawing the thumb and forefinger of the right hand down
with some considerable pressure, at the same time ensuring that the
proximal end of the tube remains undisturbed in the thorax.

Suction is applied to the other shorter tube of the underwater seal
bottle, creating a negative pressure in the bottle. The bottles are placed on the floor beneath the bed and they should never be raised above
the chest because this would cause the contents of the bottle to be
syphoned back into the thorax. A record of the drainage must be
maintained and a reading taken each hour in the first ten hours.
Any untoward haemorrhage should be reported immediately. All
these factors are important to the total care and no vital sign is considered in isolation.

It is the complete picture which enables a decision on future care
to be planned. Observation should be made every fifteen minutes
for the first hours after operation but if it is seen that a trend is developing they should be made more frequently; conversely when
the condition has become stabilised they may be made half hourly
and then hourly.

The bedside manner of the nurse should promote confidence and a serious, but reassuring manner, accompanied by a simple explanation when appropriate.

Oxygen is administered either through a Venti-mask at 28% concentration or through nasal cannulae. This is continued until the condition is stabilised.

Deep breathing exercises are commenced as soon as conciousness is regained. The physiotherapist will visit the patient and help him to cough. This is done to ensure aeration of the remaining lobes of the lung which, at this early stage, is more important than the expectoration of sputum. Passive leg exercises are commenced to avoid deep vein thrombosis.

Post operative pain is alleviated by an analgesic such as Pethidine, which does not suppress the cough reflex or produce a hypnotic effect which prevents co-operation. Adequate analgesia will enable the nurse to attend to such matters of personal hygiene and pressure area care as will be deemed necessary at this stage – remembering that the patient has been lying on the operating table for two to three hours and then on a bed with limited movement.

Provided the blood pressure is within normal limits this is the time to sit him up in bed and encourage him to pass urine. Small drinks of water may be given four to five hours after operation.

Relatives are discouraged from visiting on the first evening but the next of kin must always feel free to telephone.

On the first day after operation a light diet may be offered: if it is not taken, fluids should be encouraged. The surgeon will visit, a routine radiograph will be taken and the function of the intercostal tubes will be assessed. Provided drinks are being taken in sufficient quantity and there is no nausea or vomiting the intravenous fluids will be discontinued. The patient may sit out of bed for a short while. This will improve morale, remove weight from the buttocks and enable the lungs to expand more freely.

Physiotherapy is continued and the patient is encouraged to cough and expectorate sputum. Steam inhalations are given to facilitate the removal of tenacious sputum.

The bottles forming the underwater seal are changed daily, care being taken to clamp off the tubes prior to disconnection. Sterile bottles are used containing an agreed amount of sterile water, usually 500 ml. Any fluid in the bottles over and above this amount constitutes drainage and must be entered on the fluid balance chart.

The ambulation is increased during the next few days and there will be less necessity for strong analgesics. Pethidine injections will be replaced by oral preparations. The intercostal tubes are removed when they have ceased to function and the decision to remove them is always taken by the surgeon. The basal tube is usually removed first, about thirty-six hours after operation, and a day or so later the apical tube.

Procedure for the removal of an intercostal tube

The patient may be given a mild sedation such as 5 mg Diazepam. Two nurses are required.

A dressing trolley is prepared with the addition of tulle gras. The trolley is taken to the bedside, the procedure explained to the patient and privacy ensured. One nurse makes the patient comfortable, preferably by sitting back to front on a straight backed chair, but if necessary he may remain in bed and lean forward on a bed table. The dressing around the tube is removed and the clean nurse washes her hands. The suture securing the tube to the chest wall is cut while the second nurse supports the tube. The suction to the tube is continued and the patient instructed to take a deep breath in and hold it. The second nurse withdraws the tube as the first nurse ties the stitch to close the skin (this stitch has been left in at operation and tied only loosely in readiness for this stage). A firm tulle gras dressing is applied and the patient told to breathe normally. He is made confortable in a chair or bed. The trolley is removed from the ward together with the suction equipment.

The hazard of this procedure is that air may be introduced when the second tube is removed. This can happen if the nurses are unco-ordinated or if the patient breathes out before the seal is made on the chest wall. In any event a pneumothorax will result causing collapse of the remaining lung.

The sutures from the tube site will be removed on the third or fourth day, and the sutures from the thoracotomy wound on the tenth or twelvth day. They may be left in for an extra two days because the necessary movement and exercise of the arm may delay healing, particularly in a patient already disadvantaged because of malignant disease.

Complications following lobectomy and/or segmental resection

1. Haemorrhage
2. Prolonged air leak
3. Atelectasis or collapse of the remaining lobe
4. Effusion
5. Fistula formation
6. Empyema

1. Haemorrage. Blood stained pleural fluid is always produced after lung resection and it can be seen draining through the tubes. If it does not drain properly fibrin collects on the visceral pleura preventing free movement of the underlying lung tissue. If post operative haemorrage occurs it is seen at once filling the bottles. The blood pressure falls, the pulse rises and the patient becomes restless, sweating, cold and dyspnoeic. Any bleeding in excess of 100 ml an hour should be reported. Morphine is prescribed and a further blood transfusion is given. It may be necessary to re-open the chest, secure the bleeding point and evacuate a haemothorax.

2. Prolonged air leak may occur where the surface of the remaining lobes has been damaged. Connection to underwater seal suction is necessary to secure complete expansion of the remaining lobes until adhesion to the chest wall has been achieved or damage to the lung surface has healed.

3. Atelectasis is the term used to describe airlessness of a lobe or segment beyond an obstruction. In this case the obstruction is usually a plug of mucus which the patient failed to expectorate.

Clinical features:
a. Absence of movement on the affected side
b. Intercostal muscles appear to be sucked in on inspiration
c. Trachea and mediastinum are displaced to the affected side causing retrosternal pain, cyanosis, dyspnoea, sweating and tachycardia

The prevention of atelectasis is by encouraging breathing exercises and supervised coughing, taking care when removing intercostal tubes, and the aspiration of air and fluid as soon as it accumulates.

Treatment of atelectasis when it has occurred is by physiotherapy—energetic postural drainage, manual percussion and steam inhalations. If all these measures fail an emergency aspiration bronchoscopy must be performed.

Complete reexpansion of the remaining lobe may follow the removal of the obstruction. Alternatively re-expansion may be a slow process, taking seven to fourteen days. Rarely atelectasis may persist causing suppuration of the remaining lobes and necessitating residual pneumonectomy.

4. Effusion is demonstrated on a routine radiograph.
Clinical features:
a. Fast irregular pulse

b. Dyspnoea
c. Pyrexia

Treatment is by aspiration. The fluid must be sent to the pathological laboratory for culture and bacterial sensitivities.

5. *Fistula formation* in this sense means a communication between
the bronchial tree and the pleura. Trauma to the lung tissue may
cause an alveolar tear. This may occur during the first forty-eight
hours and is not in itself important. While the underwater seal is
attached the air will escape freely and the alveolar tissue will heal
spontaneously. If for some reason the underwater seal drainage has
been removed it is possible for a pneumonthorax to develop, causing
collapse of the underlying lung tissue. For this reason intercostal
tubes should not be removed until no bubbles can be seen. Broncho-pleural fistula may be caused by faulty suturing of the bronchial stump or by a hole which has not been seen at operation or by
infection.

Clinical features:
a. Blood-stained sputum
b. Pneumothorax is seen on chest radiograph, and possibly an effusion.

Treatment
If fluid is present a drain should be inserted and antibiotics will be
given to try to prevent or control infection because if this occurs an
empyema will develop. The hole will be sutured, which will require
the re-opening of the chest. If the underlying tissue is consolidated
or a large effusion is present it may be necessary to remove the re-
mainder of the lung.

Bronchiolar fistulae may be seen after segmented resection. They
manifest themselves immediately after operation and persist for
weeks. Infection and empyema do not necessarily follow.

Treatment
The lung is kept expanded by an underwater seal drainage and suction which must be maintained until the hole from which the leak is
originating is healed; this may take three to four weeks. Alternatively a thoracotomy may be performed and the hole sutured.

Empyema
Clinical features:
a. Malaise

b. Pyrexia

c. Anorexia

Treatment is conservative, keeping the pleura dry by repeated aspiration and the administration of antibiotics.

Nursing care after pneumonectomy is similar to that following lobectomy except in the following features.

A tube is seldom inserted to drain a pneumonectomy space. Instead the intra-pleural pressure is measured on the pneumonectomy side with a Maxwell box and is adjusted to a slightly negative level when the patient is lying supine and before leaving the theatre.

If bleeding or exudation occurs during the postoperative period it will be demonstrated on the routine radiograph and adjustment may be necessary in order to maintain the central position of the mediastinum. To avoid this some surgeons insert one tube which is attached to an underwater seal and clamped, i.e. there is no suction. This clamp is released for a short time, usually one minute in every hour. This method has also the advantage of demonstrating any post operative haemorrhage. The tube should be removed twenty-four hours after operation. The patient is nursed either on his back or on his operated side to allow full expansion of his remaining lung. Breathing exercises are commenced as soon as the patient is conscious, but only gentle coughing is encouraged under supervision because of the danger of causing a bronch-pleural fistula. Thirty-six hours are allowed to elapse before steam inhalations are given.

Complications

1. Haemorrhage
2. Effusion
3. Bronchospasm
4. Atelectasis or pneumonitis of the remaining lung
5. Broncho-pleural fistula
6. Rupture of the wound
7. Empyema

1. Because there is seldom an intercostal drain the nurse must be alert to the danger of *haemorrhage*. The source of bleeding may be from the pulmonary artery or vein, or smaller vessels. Bleeding from the large vessels is often fatal.

Clinical features:

a. Rising pulse rate with poor volume

b. Falling blood pressure
c. Restlessness
d. Pallor
e. Dyspnoea

Treatment
Morphine by injection and further transfusion. The smaller vessels may seal themselves off. If the bleeding continues it may be necessary to reopen the chest and tie off the bleeding points again.

2. Effusion: as for lobectomy.

3. Bronchospasm. This may occur during the first post operative week and must be recognised and treated quickly.

Clinical features:
a. Severe distress
b. Breathlessness due to lack of oxygen

Treatment
The administration of Salbutamol or similar bronchodilators, by injection, and Salbutamol by nebulizer three times a day. Cortocosteroids may be used.

4. Altelectasis of the remaining lung constitutes a surgical emergency and requires immediate bronchoscopy.

5. Bronchopleural fistula is life threatening following pneumonectomy.
Clinical features:
a. Blood stained sputum
b. Tachycardia
c. Pleural fluid may be expectorated

Treatment
Lie the patient on the operated side to prevent fluid entering the remaining lung. The stump needs to be resutured as soon as possible to avoid an empyema.

5. Rupture of the wound: same as after lobectomy.

6. Empyema: same as after lobectomy.

Radiotherapy

A small number of cases are suitable for *curative* radiotherapy.

These are usually patients who are operable from the surgical point of view, but whose general condition precludes operation. They include patients with chronic bronchitis or heart failure who develop a bronchial carcinoma Curative radiotherapy can also be used as the main form of treatment when the tumour is small but situated in the trachea or one of the main bronchi, so that surgical removal is impossible. *Palliative* radiotherapy is valuable in alleviating symptoms which arise in those cases which are inoperable and too advanced for curative radiotherapy.

Radiotherapy is of particular value where the tumour or secondary glands press on the great veins returning blood to the heart from the upper limbs, head and neck (*superior vena caval obstruction*). These patients feel very uncomfortable, having a swollen face and arms and a constant feeling that they are being asphyxiated.

Prior to treatment the patient's general condition will be checked by doing a full blood count, haemoglobin, white cell count, platelets urea and electrolytes. All patients anticipating treatment by radiotherapy will suffer some degree of depression: this may manifest itself by withdrawal or conversely aggresive behaviour or by apparent euphoria. These symptoms are dealt with as they occur but they are minimised by attentive nursing care where there is time to talk through the patient's fears with him. There is a general ignorance and mystique about radiotherapy and a simple explanation is necessary. Continual re-assurance is essential for all patients and this can be ensured by maintaining a good rapport between nurse and patient.

Attendance is required in the radiotherapy department daily for four to six weeks for curative radiotherapy and for one to two weeks for palliative radiotherapy.

Symptoms associated with treatment by radiotherapy

a. Anorexia and nausea. These symptoms may be present prior to treatment or they may be exacerbated by the patient's expectations of the treatment. The toxic effects of radiation on tissue and the breakdown of rapidly dividing cells are physiological factors which may cause anorexia and nausea. The patient may be receiving drugs such as Digoxin which may cause vomiting.

A bland high protein diet with milk supplements should be encouraged and there are plenty of propriety preparations available to promote variety.

b. Tiredness. This is most marked when the brain is being irradiated. The other factor which may cause tiredness is the travelling involved as mentioned above. Regular and adequate rest should be encouraged. The patient should be warned that it may occur and that it is a normal reaction.

c. Dry, irritating cough. This is caused by inflammation to the mucosa of the trachea and bronchial tree and can be treated with linctus.

d. Dysphagia. This occurs for the same reason and can be treated with Mucaine Suspension.

e. Pneumonitis. This occurs a few weeks after the course of treatment and presents with breathlessness, a productive cough and superimposed infection. Antibiotics and a small dose of Prednisolone are prescribed and steam inhalations are given.

f. Acute pulmonary fibrosis. Pneumonitis may progress to permanent pulmonary fibrosis causing a marked reduction in the functioning lung tissue. If the patient's respiratory function was already impaired by chronic lung disease this further development could seriously limit his exercise tolerance.

g. Skin problems. The largest dose of radiation falls on the skin and as the rays travel further into the tissue the dose diminishes. It follows therefore that some redness and tenderness will be experienced over the irradiated areas during the course of treatment. Instructions should be given to keep the area dry and avoid washing it. Creams and ointments should not be applied unless they are prescribed by the radiotherapist or his staff. The area should be protected from extremes of temperature, sunlight or cold wind. Most patients do not need any particular treatment to their skin. They complain of irritation for which baby powder, which does not contain zinc or bismuth, may be prescribed. Desquamation sometimes occurs in the axilla as a result of sweating; if there is no infection it can be left until healing takes place and the new epidermis is formed. In the presence of infection an antiseptic ointment, such as Cetrimide, may be prescribed.

There is often no need to hospitalise a patient receiving a short course of palliative radiotherapy, which always gives him hope and a sense of purpose.

Chemotherapy

The idea of treating lung cancer with drugs is very attractive. Surgery and radiotherapy treat specific areas of malignant tissue by selecting that area only for attention and if secondary deposits or minute areas of growth have been left untreated inadvertently, then recurrence is the rule. In theory it would be far more efficient to use a selective agent which would seek out all the cancer cells in the body and leave the normal cells to continue their development. This is not yet possible but cytotoxic drugs are being used increasingly in the treatment of all types of cancer. They work by interfering with the development of protein in the cells at different stages in their cycle according to the drug employed.

The results of cytotoxic chemotherapy in the treatment of lung cancer have been disappointing and the most we have learnt to expect at this stage is palliation. Oat cell carcinoma is more susceptible to treatment than squamous cell or adenocarcinoma. Broadly speaking there are three methods by which the drugs can be used:

1. One drug over a period of days, given either orally or intravenously
2. Multiple drugs in one large dose
3. Instillation into the pleural space

It is the prerogative of the physician to select the drugs and method of administration and he will take the following factors into consideration:

a. The particular cancer cell that he is going to treat
b. The margin between the therapeutic dose and the toxic dose
c. The time required for the recovery of normal cells before the next treatment
d. The side effect of each drug—the most serious of which is bone marrow depression causing leukopenia and bleeding
e. Liver and renal function—because most of the drugs are metabolised in the liver and excreted by the kidneys

The administration of cytotoxic therapy produces stress in the patient and the nurse must be able to support her patient. This means she must make the following assessments:

Mental state. Is the personality stable? Are the relationships with family and friends such that they will help him through his treatment? Fear and depression are very understandable in malignant disease. The administration of Methotrexate can exacerbate the de-

Table Cytotoxic drugs in common use in thoracic medical units

Preparation	Mode of action	Route	Side effects	Nursing watchpoints
Antimetabolities (agents that fall into this group are most effective at the beginning of the cell cycle)				
Methotrexate	Toxic to liver and kidney if used in high doses	I.V. or I.M.	Bone marrow depression Stomatitis Gastro intestinal disturbances Skin rash Cystitis	Alert to infection and bleeding Frequent oral hygiene Light easily digested diet Apply calamine lotion Adequate fluids Deteriorates in sunlight – Cover bottle with dark bag
Alkylating agents (action takes place during any stage of the cell's life cycle)				
Cyclophosphamide (Endoxana)	Excreated via the kidneys Immunosuppressant	I.V. or Oral	Bone marrow depression Stomatitis Nausea and vomiting Alopecia Cystitis Alteration in taste	Alert to infection and bleeding Frequent oral hygiene Light easily digested diet Arrange for wig fitting Adequate fluids Give some foods with decisive flavours
Bisulphan (Myleran)	Cummulative effect White cell count slow to recover or does not recover at all Excreted via the kidneys	Oral	Bone marrow depression Gynaecomastia (male breast enlargement) Amenorrhoea Pigmentation of skin Irreversible pulmonary fibrosis	Alert to infection and bleeding Warn the patient Steroids are prescribed
Chlorambucil (Leukeran)	Slow to act	Oral	Bone marrow depression Nausea and vomiting	Alert to infection and bleeding

Drug	Route	Pharmacology	Side effects	Nursing care
	Intra pleural		Nausea	bleeding Light easily digested diet Great care needed to ensure no solution touches eyes or skin
Thiotepa	I.V.	Cummulative effect	Bone marrow depression Nausea and vomiting Headache pyrexia Gastro intestinal perforation Mild anaemia	Alert to infection and bleeding Light easily digested diet Fluids, temperature check Watch for abdominal pain
Natural products				
Vinblastine	I.V.	Leukopenia, particularly in jaundiced patients	Bone marrow depression Nausea and vomiting Peripheral neuritis Headache Vertigo Constipation Circulatory failure	Alert to infection and bleeding Light easily digested diet Alert to numbness of limbs Mild aperients
Vincristine	I.V.	Metabolised by the liver Neurotoxic	Stomatitis Nausea and vomiting Abdominal pain Constipation Dysuria Peripheral neuritis	Frequent oral hygiene Light easily digested diet Mild aperients Adequate fluids Report complaints of numbness of limbs or unusual gait.
Natulan	Oral	Metabolised by the liver Excreted by the kidneys		

pression through Prednisolone may go some way towards relieving it.

Weight. It is necessary to know the weight before treatment can be prescribed. Skin lesions will not heal readily whilst immunosuppressive drugs are being used and a low white cell count may give rise to infection.

Oral hygiene. This needs to be meticulous. The mouth should be inspected with a torch. Ill fitting dentures, mouth ulcers, or broken teeth should be corrected before the commencement of treatment.

Mobility. Before becoming breathless should be noted as this is a good guide to general condition and can be used as a base line to measure the effectiveness of treatment.

Oral administration of anti-neoplastic agents can be monitored by routine blood checks and the routine observation of the patient.

Administration by the intravenous route requires very careful nursing care by experienced staff. The local protocol in checking and administering drugs must be observed in every detail. Some drugs are given by syringe–i.e. cyclophosphamide 250 mg daily for five days, and some are given in solution and many are introduced into a ready established I.V. infusion at a specific rate, sometimes in conjunction with a volumetric infusion pump. It is very important to ensure that the prescribed rate is adhered to. If it is too fast the patient is not only at risk from too high a dose of the drug, causing unnecessary toxic side effects, but he is also in danger because his circulation becomes overloaded, with the risk of congestive cardiac failure developing. Extravasation of the infusion may cause severe local damage. The physician must be notified immediately so that the treatment may be re-established without delay and the blood level of the drug maintained.

Table at the end of this chapter sets out clearly the data required by the nurse, including the complications which may arise associated with each preparation. It will be seen that infection and bleeding from bone marrow depression and nausea and vomiting are common concomitants of this method of treatment, for which the caring team will develop management skills. Nausea and vomiting can be minimised by the administration of Chlorpromazine one hour before treatment commences. Unfortunately there is some debate that this practice may reduce the therapeutic effect of the drugs.

In any event severe vomiting is frustrating and uncomfortable for the patient and may seriously effect the fluid and electrolyte balance. The bone marrow depression is monitored carefully between treatments and the blood count allowed to return to acceptable levels before the next treatment is commenced.

Alopecia is the longest lasting and most distressing side effect of cyclophosphamide and the patient needs explanation and reassurance before treatment is begun. It is truthful to say that the hair may fall out but given time it will grow again. Arrangements should be made for a wig or, if at all possible, a visit may be made to a department store where one can be selected with the aid of a close friend or relative.

Anti-neoplastic agents, commonly cyclophosphamide or mustine, may be instilled into the pleural space in the treatment of malignant pleural effusion. The pleural space is aspirated daily until it is as dry as possible. At the end of the procedure the drug is introduced and the needle withdrawn. This is an effective palliative measure reducing or abolishing the need for frequent chest aspiration.

Other tumours of the lung

Other tumours of the lung are relatively rare in comparison with bronchial carcinoma. *Alveolar cell carcinoma* arises in the alveoli and grows along the alveolar walls. One or both lungs are involved, and curative resection is not possible.

Secondary tumours of the lung are common. The X-ray appearance is frequently characteristic and may appear as a single 'cannonball' or as multiple nodules or miliary mottling known as *lymphangitis carcinomatosis*.

Benign tumours can be made up of fibrous tissue (*fibroma*), fatty tissue (*lipoma*) or cartilage (*hamartoma*). None of these tumours has any special characteristic which can lead to easy identification. In all cases thoracotomy and resection is necessary in case the X-ray shadow is really due to a bronchial carcinoma.

A number of tumours arise in the mediastinum and show on the X-ray as a mass between the lungs (Fig. 6.14). These can include benign and malignant growths of the thymus and thyroid glands, Hodgkin's disease of the glands of the mediastinum, and lymphosarcomas. Diagnosis can only be made by taking a biopsy.

Tumours of the ribs cause pain and show on an X-ray as a shadow extending from the rib. They may be benign (*chondroma*) or

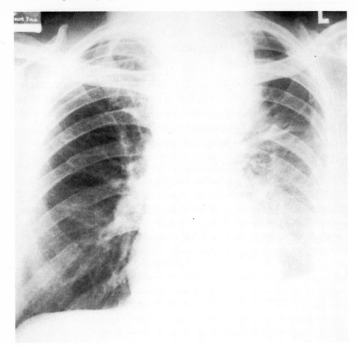

Fig. 6.14 An X-ray showing a tumour in the mediastinum

malignant (*sarcoma*). Secondary deposits from cancers elsewhere in the body frequently occur in the ribs – especially from the prostate gland.

Seven
Diseases of the pleura and diaphragm

Pleurisy

We have already seen that the pleura, the membrane which covers the lung and which also lines the interior of the chest wall (p. 11) can be involved by malignant invasion from a lung cancer. Other diseases also affect the pleura and usually reach it from the surrounding structures. Most commonly the lung is the source. Pleurisy occurs in various forms:

a. *Dry pleurisy*
b. *Pleurisy with effusion* (or wet pleurisy)
c. *Empyema*

Dry pleurisy

This consists of an inflammation or irritation of the pleural membrane. The movement of respiration and the consequent rubbing together of the pleural surfaces causes a characteristic pain on deep breathing.

Any disease in the lung may develop near the pleural surface and cause dry pleurisy. The common disorders producing this condition are: pneumonia, lung abscess, tuberculosis, pulmonary infarction and injury to the chest wall.

Treatment is essentially that of the underlying cause. Pain may be relieved by the administration of analgesic drugs. The correct position in bed is the one which is most comfortable for the patient. Many find it better to lie on the affected side since this diminishes movement of that side of the chest.

Alternatively a semi-recumbent position with the affected side well supported by pillows gives relief from pain. Whilst nursing the patient it should be appreciated that rotation of the trunk and side to side movements exacerbate the pain.

Pleurisy with effusion

Clear, sterile fluid may develop in the pleural space in a number of conditions:

Inflammations: a. pneumonia.
　　　　　　　b. lung abscess.
　　　　　　　c. bronchiectasis.
　　　　　　　d. tuberculosis.

Mechanical: a. heart disease.
　　　　　　b. diseases of the kidney, such as nephritis.
　　　　　　c. leukaemia.
　　　　　　d. penetrating wounds of the chest.

Sympathetic: a. from pus under the diaphragm (subphrenic abscess).

Neoplastic: a. a primary or secondary lung cancer.
　　　　　　b. pleural mesothelioma.

On a chest X-ray the fluid appears as a dense uniform shadow on the affected side (Fig. 7.1). Proof of the presence of pleural fluid is

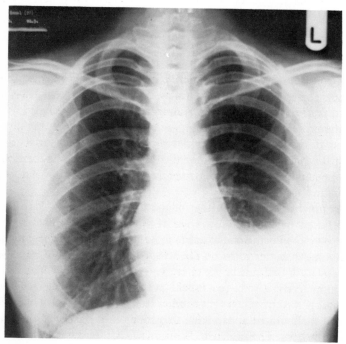

Fig. 7.1 An X-ray showing a moderate pleural effusion

given by aspiration of the pleural cavity as described above. Some of the aspirated fluid is placed in a small sterile bottle to be sent to the laboratory.

The treatment of a pleural effusion is that of the primary cause. In effusions which result from inflammation, the chest is aspirated (using a syringe, two-way tap and needle) until no more fluid can be obtained. The aspirating needle is then left in the chest with the tap turned off so that no air can be sucked into the pleural cavity. Another syringe containing a solution of the appropriate antibiotic is then attached to the tap and injected.

The inhalation of asbestos can cause a tumour known as a *mesothelioma*. The hazard from asbestos is much more widespread that has been appreciated, and even a very minor exposure to the dust (such as living near an asbestos factory or handling the dusty clothes of an asbestos worker) can cause the development of this growth. In addition, the tumour may not develop until up to forty years later.

The tumour produces a large effusion which always recurs after aspiration. The diagnosis is made by pleural biopsy. Curative treatment is impossible, but cytotoxic drugs are useful for palliative purposes.

Empyema

When the fluid in the pleural cavity is found to be purulent, rather than amber or straw-coloured, the patient is said to have an *empyema*, or localized collection of pus in the pleural cavity.

The most common cause of an empyema is the extension of bacterial infection from the lung, usually from a pneumonia or a lung abscess. Infection can also reach the pleura from a penetrating chest wound. It can also be a complication of thoracic surgery, and may result from spread of infection through the diaphragm from a subphrenic abscess.

Where the infection follows pneumonia, it ususally develops one to two weeks later. The temperature which had fallen starts to rise again, and the patient looks ill, sweats, and complains of tiredness and loss of appetite. The white cell count of the blood is raised, and the chest X-ray shows the usual appearance of a pleural effusion. Aspiration produces a turbid fluid full of polymorphs, and bacterial culture will show the causative organism. The patient is propped up on pillows. The infected effusion is aspirated daily to keep the pleural cavity as dry as possible. The appropriate antibiotic is injected into the cavity after the aspiration and is also given systema-

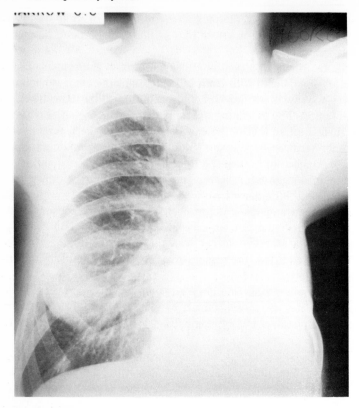

Fig 7.2 An X-ray showing right thoraplasty

tically (by mouth or by intramuscular injection). This treatment may resolve the empyema.

Where daily aspiration is not successful, surgical drainage must be carried out. A portion of a rib near the lowest part of the empyema cavity is cut away, and a drainage tube is inserted into the bottom of the cavity so that efficient drainage can occur. The drainage tube is usually connected to an underwater seal. It is necessary to do a rib resection because the empyema tube will be in situ for an extended period; frequently several weeks. Without a rib resection there is increased risk of pain and infection, pain because the nerve of the superior rib is put under stress, infection because the organisms from the empyema space will invade the wound. When the rib has been resected there is sufficient space for the soft tissue to envelope the tube without compressing the nerve. Deep breathing and movement should be encouraged to expand the underlying lung and obliterate the empyema space.

Deep breathing will also prevent the chest wall becoming fixed by the development of dense fibrous tissue. Close observation is necessary to see that the tube does not become blocked, and the colour and amount of fluid draining into the bottle every 24 hours must be recorded. Antibiotic treatment continues both systematically and into the pleural space. The antibiotic chosen depends on the causative organisms.

The nursing care for a patient with an empyema tube is similar to that of an intercostal tube except in the following points:

1. The largest tube available is used because this enables free drainage of purulent viscous material.
2. Care must be taken to ensure that the empyema tube does not come out of the empyema and merely lodge in the chest wall.
3. The tube remains in situ as long as the drainage persists and until the empyema space is obliterated.
4. When the drainage is less than 100 ml a day the tube could be attached to a small plastic container allowing greater mobility for the patient. When there is enough adhesion of lung to the chest wall the tube may be cut and allowed to drain into a dressing. It is possible that the patient may be discharged to the care of the general practitioner and the district nurse.
5. A sinogram should follow at two weekly intervals until occlusion has been achieved.

In some patients the empyema cavity will not close, owing to the undue thickness of its walls. In these cases, the thickened covering is removed by the operation of *decortication*. The chest is opened and the thick membrane covering the lung is incised down to the pleura. A layer of cleavage is found between the empyema wall and the normal pleura, and the surgeon can then peel this thick membrane off the lung. In cases where the empyema wall will not strip off the pleura, *thoracoplasty* may be necessary. In this operation portions of rib are removed so that the whole of the chest wall falls in to meet the visceral pleura (Fig. 7.2).

Haemothorax

The term *haemothorax* is applied to the presence of blood in the pleural cavity. It usually follows injury to the chest wall or a thoracic operation, and may complicate a spontaneous pneumothorax (see p. 134).

If the bleeding is copious and rapid, the patient will be shocked and collapsed with rapid pulse and respiration. There are signs of fluid in the chest, and the diagnosis is confirmed by aspiration of blood from the pleural cavity. Aspiration is always possible, since blood in the pleural cavity does not clot. The constant movement of the lung in breathing agitates the blood and leads to its *fibrin* (the material in blood which forms the clot), separating out and being deposited on the pleural surface of the lung to form a thick membrane. The resulting defibrinated blood cannot clot.

The patient must be kept quietly at rest and lying flat. He is given oxygen via a polymask. Vital signs must be observed and recorded quarter hourly. A blood transfusion may be required, so the nurse must get the appropriate trolley ready. The bloody fluid is aspirated, and the pleural space kept as dry as possible by further daily aspiration. Antibiotics are given to prevent any infection occurring (since blood makes a good culture medium for bacteria). Where bleeding continues the chest must be opened and the bleeding points tied off, or where the space cannot be obliterated, decortication must be carried out (see p. 134).

Spontaneous pneumothorax

The term *pneumothorax* means that there is air in the pleural cavity

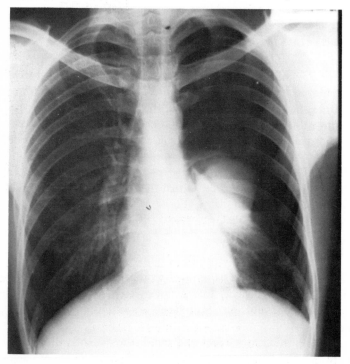

Fig. 7.3 An X-ray showing a spontaneous pneumothorax

(Fig. 7.3). Normally this potential space between the visceral and parietal layers of the pleura contains only a little lubricating fluid. Air can enter the space from outside as a result of a penetrating wound of the chest, or it can be deliberately inserted through a needle for diagnostic or therapeutic purposes. More commonly, however, a pneumothorax arises when a small *bulla* (air space) beneath the visceral pleura ruptures outwards. This often happens in apparently healthy young people, particularly when they are taking violent exercise or engaging in underwater diving. A less frequent cause these days is the rupture of a small tuberculous focus underneath the visceral pleura or the rupture of a lung abscess. In the latter case pus will also form in the pleural space — a *pyopneumothorax* (Fig. 7.4).

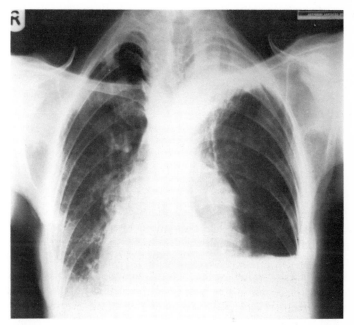

Fig. 7.4 An X-ray showing a pyoneumothorax

Usually the hole in the pleura closes as the lung collapses. In some cases, however, the hole in the lung is held open. The air may either flow in and out or be trapped by a valve mechanism, so that the pressure within the chest cavity steadily builds up after each breath (Fig. 7.5). The latter condition is called a *tension pneumothorax* and causes compression of the heart and the great vessels, so death may occur unless the pressure is relieved.

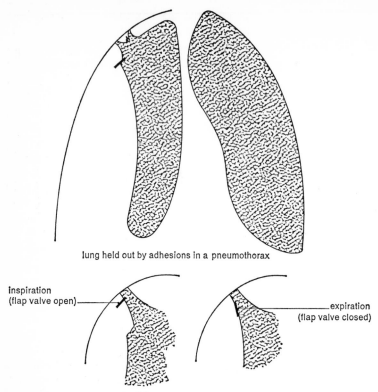

lung held out by adhesions in a pneumothorax

Inspiration
(flap valve open)

expiration
(flap valve closed)

Fig. 7.5 A tension pneumothorax

The patient will commonly feel shortness of breath and pain on the side of the lesion. When that side is tapped with a finger, the chest sounds hollow and no breath sounds can be heard. An X-ray is diagnostic. A non-tension pneumothorax usually absorbs slowly, but it may take many weeks before the lung is fully expanded. Often, therefore, air is aspirated from the pleural cavity daily using a pneumothorax apparatus. About 600 cc of air are removed on each occasion, the amount being controlled by the intrapleural pressure. Usually the final pressure after removal of air should be around 8 cm of water on inspiration, and 4 cm on expiration.

There are several types of pneumothorax apparatus. The most common is that of Morland, and another type is that of Lillingston and Pearson (Fig. 7.6).

Where there is a tension pneumothorax, a rubber intercostal catheter is placed between the ribs into the pleural space (via a trocher and cannula) and connected to an underwater drain. When air has stopped bubbling through the underwater drain for 24

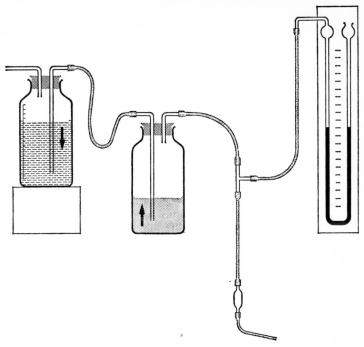

Fig. 7.6 The Lillingston and Pearson pneumothorax apparatus. Water, flowing from the left-hand (upper) bottle to that on the right, displaces air, which is then driven via hollow tubing and a cottonwool filler to the needle in the patient's chest. A side tube leads to a water manometer. Reversal of the bottles enables air to be withdrawn from the chest.

hours, the catheter is clipped off and an X-ray is taken. If, after a further 24 hours, air has not re-accumulated in the pleural space, then the intercostal catheter can be removed.

Occasionally, when the underlying lung is full of bullae caused by emphysema, the surgeon inserts a telescope into the pleural cavity under a local or general anaesthetic and explores the lung surface (*thoracoscopy*). If he can see the hole in the lung, he inserts another cannula into the chest and through this he passes a long probe. He applies silver nitrate to the hole in the lung to help healing and promote closure. Very rarely, a lobectomy may be necessary.

Recurrence is extremely common with a pneumothorax. When this has occurred on two further occasions, the surgeon often induces an adhesive pleuritis, either by putting 10 ml of 1 per cent silver nitrate into the pleural cavity or by dusting talc containing a little iodine over the surface of the lung through a cannula inserted into the chest. More commonly pleurectomy is carried out. In this operation the parietal pleura is stripped from the chest wall and the upper mediastinum so as to leave a raw surface to which the visceral pleura can then adhere, which secures the permanent expansion of the lung.

The patient returns from theatre with an intercostal tube on the affected side. This is attached to suction apparatus. There is some post operative pain resulting from the pleurisy and analgesics should be administered. Deep breathing can be encouraged. A daily radiograph will be taken to monitor the lung expansion. Pyrexia can be expected on the second or third day which signifies that the pleurisy is present and adhesions are forming. Antibiotics are not prescribed because this would interfere with the infective process which, in this case, is desirable. When the lung has been fully expanded for twenty-four hours the suction may be discontinued and the intercostal tube removed.

Diseases of the diaphragm

Hiccup

Recurrent spasm of the diaphragm leads to an involuntary expulsion of air from the lungs with a characteristic sound called a *hiccup*. In rare cases, this may be so prolonged that it interferes with eating and sleeping and, in the elderly, it may lead to extreme exhaustion.

It can be due to a variety of causes:

a. *Alimentary*: from irritation of the oesophagus or stomach by overeating or from spices and pickles, intestinal obstruction, inflammation of the peritoneum;
b. *Nervous*: hysteria, cerebral tumour;
c. *Local Irritation*: from the pressure of enlarged thoracic lymph nodes or a pericardal effusion, or from inflammation of the pleura over the upper surface of the diaphragm;
d. *Uraemia*: for details of this see the companion volume in this series, *The Urological System*.

Simple hiccup can often be relieved by holding the breath, by pressure on the chest or by inhaling 5 per cent carbon dioxide in oxygen. In more severe cases, an intramuscular injection of 50 mg of chlorpromazine may be required.

Hiccup due to organic disease or to local irritation is only relieved by removal of the cause. Thus peritonitis may need excision of an inflamed appendix and drainage of the peritoneal cavity.

Hernia

The diaphragm is made up from several masses of tissue which may not always join together correctly. In these cases there is a defect in the muscle sheet separating the thorax from the peritoneal cavity. Since such a hole in the diaphragm is covered only by pleura and peritoneum, parts of the stomach or intestine can make their way through it. The hernia may be noted on routine X-rays, and sometimes gives difficulty in the differential diagnosis of symptomless shadows in the chest. It is unlikely to produce respiratory symptoms, but may give rise to abdominal ones — for instance, the pain characteristic of *hiatus hernia*.

Further reading

Reference book

Crofton, J. & Douglas, A. (1981) *Respiratory Diseases* 3rd edition. Edinburgh Blackwell.

General books

Belcher, J.R. & Sturridge (1972) *Thoracic Surgical Mangement* 4th edition London, Bailliere Tindall.

Caplin, M. (1980) *The Tuberculin Test in Clinical Practise* London, Bailliere Tindall.

Collins, J.V. (1979) *A Synopsis of Chest Disease* London, J. Wright.

Comroe, J.H. (1974) *Physiology of Respiration* 2nd edition Chicago, Year Book Medical Publishers.

Gaskell, D.V. & Webber, B.A. (1977) *The Brompton Hospital Guide to Chest Physiotherapy* 3rd edition Oxford, Blackwell.

Goodfield, R. & Spalding, J.M.K. (1976) *A Nurse's Guide to Artificial Ventilation* London, Arnold E.

Henley, A. (1980) *Asian Patients in Hospital and at Home* London, King Edward Hospital Fund for London.

Ross, J.D. & Horne, N.W. *Modern Drug Treatment in Tuberculosis* London, Chest Heart and Stroke Association.

Walter, J. (1977) *Cancer and Radiotherapy* 2nd edition Edinburgh, Churchill Livingstone.

Articles

Cassall, S.J. (1979) Patient on a Ventilator. *Nursing Mirror*, **148** 4.

Grenville-Mathers, R. (1977) Cor Pulmonale 2 3 *Chest Heart and Stroke Journal*

Kiely, T. (1980) Clinical Care of a Child with Pneumonia and a Detailed Nursing Plan *Nursing Mirror* **150,** 96.

Nursing Journal of Clinical Nursing (1979)   6 Breathing Part 1 (Sept)
                                               7 Breathing Part II (Nov)
                                                  Medical Education
                                                  (International) Ltd

Thomas, S. (1979) Observation and Charting of Respiration *Nursing Mirror* **148** 24.

Tym, G. (1980) Obstructive Airway Disease in Children *Nursing Mirror* **150** (27 March) 18, (3 April): 36, (10 April) : 32, (17 April): 26, (24 April): 25.

Webb, K. & Mitchell, D. (1979) Sarcoidosis. Clinical Presentation Diagnosis Investigation and Treatment *Nursing Mirror* **149** 44.

Index

Abdominal breathing, 10
Accessory muscles, 10, 12, 59, 60, 61, 65
Acid fast bacilli, 75
A.C.T.H., 63
Acute infections, 30
Adenocarcinoma, 101
Adrenaline, 62, 66
Adult TB disease, 80
Aerosols, 62
Air hunger, 25
Air leak, 117
Alcoban, 44
Allergens, 60, 64
Allergy desensitisation, 66
Allergy testing, 65
Alopecia, 127
Alveolar cell carcinoma, 127
Alveolar membrane, 47
Alveoli, 3, 5, 11, 14, 19, 47, 64, 76, 125
Aminophylline, 32, 39, 40, 42, 51, 53, 63
Amoxycillin, 32, 39, 51
Ampicillin, 50
Analgesics, 26, 129
Antibiotics, 39, 44, 64, 81, 90
Artery
  carotid, 1, 14
  innominate, 1
  intercostal, 8
  pulmonary, 1, 11
  subclavian, 1
Articular process, 6
Asbestosis, 97, 100, 131
Aspergillosis, 43
Asphyxia, 14
Asthma, 28, 45, 59, 68, 90
Atmospheric, pollution 6
Atalectasis, 42, 103, 104, 117
Atypical pneumonia, 40

Barnes respirator, 63
Barrier nursing, 85

BCG vaccination, 84, 95
Becotide, 62
Benign tumours, 125
Benzyl penicillin, 39
Bird respirator, 6
Bisulphan, 124
Byssinosis, 77
B.L.B. mask, 65
Blood stream
  function of, 1
  spread of infection, 79
Brain, 13
  respiratory centre, 13, 51
  tumour, 106, 138
Breathing exercises, 50, 54, 115
Bricanyl, 62
Bronchi, 3
Bronchial buds, 4
Bronchial carcinoma, 26, 27, 70, 72, 90, 92–100, 102, 103
Bronchial lavage, 54
Bronchiectasis, 89
  sicca 91
Bronchiolar fistula, 118
Bronchioles, 12
Bronchitis, 30
Bronchitis and emphysema, 45
Bronchography, 91, 92
Bronchogenic tuberculosis, 80
Broncho pleural fistula, 120
Broncho pneumonia, 34, 41, 90
Bronchoscopy, 69, 72, 106
Bronchospasm, 33, 120
Bullae, 47, 48, 134

Calcification, 77
Cancer of breast, 98
Candida albicans, 44
Carbolfuchsin, 75
Carbon dioxide, 2, 11, 13, 14, 19, 50
Carbon monoxide, 14
Carina of the bronchi, 3
Cardiac catheterisation, 20

Carotid artery, 14
Carotid sinus, 14
Caseous area, 76
Central tendon, 8
Cerebral abscess, 73
Cervical rib, 7
Chemical control of breathing, 13–14
Chemotherapy, 87, 123
Chest aspiration, 110, 111, 132
Cheyne-Stokes respiration, 25
Chlorambucil, 124
Chondroma, 127
Chromates, 100
Chronic bronchitis, 45
Cilia, 4, 5, 30, 46, 90
Clavicle, 6, 10
Clubbing of fingers, 28, 91
Collapse therapy, 88
Columnar epithelium, 4
Complications of tuberculosis, 81
Congestive cardiac failure, 47, 53
Control of breathing, 12–14
Corticosteroids, 63
Cough, 21, 23, 31, 68–70, 81, 90, 113, 115
Cushing's syndrome, 105
Cyanide, 14
Cyanosis, 41, 57, 64
Cyclophosphamide, 112
Cycloserine, 88
Cyst, 70
Cytotoxic drugs, 124, 125

Decortication, 133, 138
Deformities of the chest, 28
Dermatophagoids, 60
Diabetes, 24
Diaphragm, 5, 8–10, 12, 54, 112, 138
Diazepam, 64
Digoxin, 53
Dilation of bronchial tubes, 88, 89
Dionosil, 91
District Community Physician, 89
Dorsal vertebrae, 6
Dry pleurisy, 129
Dyspnoea, 21, 24, 81, 97, 103

Edinburgh mask, 51
Effusion, 117
Emotional disorders, 26, 61, 67
Emphysema, 47, 53, 61, 157
Empyema, 70, 117, 129, 193
Endoxana, 124
Eosinophil cells, 61
Epiglottis, 3
Erythema nodosum, 94
Erythromycin, 44

Ethambutol, 87
Ethionamide, 88
Examination tray, 27
Expectorants, 23
Expiration, 2, 12, 13, 49, 54–56
Expiratory reserve capacity, 16
Extrinsic asthma, 60
Exudative lesions, 76, 77

Facial palsy, 94
Feather pillows, 65
Fever, 81, 93
Fibre-optic bronchoscopy, 108
Fibroma, 127
Fluocytosine, 44
Fetus, 3
Forced expiratory volume, 17, 49
Forced vital capacity, 15, 49
Foreign bodies, 68
Friar's balsam, 40
Freidlander's pneumonia, 36
Frusemide, 53

Gas exchange, 15, 19–20
Gastric lavage, 82
Geiger counter, 19
Glottis, oedema of, 107
Grass pollens, 65
Gynaecomastia, 105

Haematemesis, 23
Haemoglobin, 11, 14, 112
Haemophilus influenzae, 32–47
Haemoptysis, 23–24, 81, 91, 103, 107
Haemothorax, 133
Hamartoma, 127
Heaf gun, 83
Heart 5, 135
  diseases of, 26
  failure, 25, 28, 47, 53, 55, 121
Hernia, 139
Herpes simplex, 34
Hiatus hernia, 36, 124
Hiccup, 138
Hilar glands, 95, 103
Hilum, 102
Histamine, 60
Hodgkin's disease, 125
Horner's syndrome, 105
House dust, 60, 65, 75
House mite, 60
Hydrocortisone, 63
Hysteria, 138

Industrial asthma, 60
Influenza, 50, 90
Infundibulum, 4

Inhalation of tubercle bacilli, 75
Ingestion of tubercle bacilli, 76
Inspiration, 12, 13, 49, 60
Inspiratory reserve capacity, 16
Intercostal drainage, 136
Intercostal artery, 8
Intercostal muscle, 7, 8, 10, 12
Intercostal tube, 116
Intrinsic asthma, 59
Investigation of patient, 27–29
Iodine, 91, 92
Isoniazid, 87, 88
Isoprenaline, 53

Kidneys, 79, 81, 130
Kweim test, 95
Kyphosis, 28

Laryngeal swab, 82
Laryngo-tracheal groove, 4
Larynx, 2, 3, 105, 107
Legionnaire's disease, 36
Leukaemia, 130
Lillington and Pearson pneumothorax
   apparatus, 135
Lipoma, 127
Lobar pneumonia, 33–36, 81
   treatment, 37
Lobectomy, 112
Lobes of lungs, 1, 4, 11, 72, 89, 92, 93,
   103, 110
Loss of weight, 21, 27, 81, 94, 103
Löwenstein's medium, 75
Lung, 1–5, 10–12, 15, 47, 49, 60, 62,
   69, 78–80, 89, 90, 93, 99, 109,
   110, 112, 123, 125, 129–133,
   134–138
   abscess, 23, 69–73, 104, 134
   cancer, 23, 98–124, 130
   cancer investigation of, 106–109
   cancer treatment of, 111–123
Lymphangitis carcinomatosis, 125, 127
Lymphatic duct, 79
Lymphatics, 79
Lymph glands, 94, 95
Lymph nodes, 79
Lymphosarcoma, 128

Malignant tumours, 125
Mantoux test, 83
Manubrium, 6
Mass radiography units, 76
Measles, 4, 90
Mediastinum, 11, 105, 126
Medical Research Council Unit, 85
Medihaler, Iso, 62
Medulla oblongata, 13

Meningitis, 79, 80
Mesothelioma, 131
Methotrexate, 124
Miliary tuberculosis, 79–81
Mogadon, 53
Moniliasis, 44
Morland pneumonthorax apparatus, 135
Morphine, 39, 64
Mucus, 39, 57, 60, 61, 70
Mycetoma, 44
Mycobacterium tuberculosis, 74

Nasal polyps, 67
Natulan, 124
Neck, 79
Nervous control of breathing, 13
Nitrogen, 19
Nitrogen mustard, 19
Nystatin, 44

Oat cell tumour, 101
Obstruction of bronchial tree, 45
Oedema, 49
Oesophagus, 23, 105, 138
Oxygen, 1, 11, 14, 19, 37–39, 51, 64,
   65, 107, 131
Oxymeter, 20

Pain in the chest, 21–25, 81, 103
Palate, 3
Palpating the chest, 28
Pancoast tumour, 105
Parietal pleura, 11
Parietal space, 11
Parotid glands, 94
Paroxsymal nocturnal dyspnoea, 23
Parrot – Gohn focus, 78
Pasteurisation of milk, 75, 76, 84
Pavement epithelium, 11
Peak expiratory flow rate (PEFR), 17,
   49
Pectoralis major, 10
Penicillin, 67
Percussing the chest, 28
Peritoneum, 138, 139
Pethidine, 39, 115
Pets, 65
Peyer's patches, 79
Pharynx, 2, 3
Phenergan, 64
Phrenic nerves, 10
Physiotherapy, 115
Phyllocontin, 62
Pleura, 11, 24, 33, 70, 102, 107, 129,
   138
Pleural biopsy, 109, 110
Pleural effusion, 81, 104, 109, 125

Pleural membrane, 129
Pleural mesothelioma, 131
Pleurisy, 24–25, 70, 81, 129–138
Pneumococcal pneumonia, *see* Lobar
    pneumonia
Pneumonococcus, 33, 47
Pneumoconiosis, 97
Pneumonectomy, 112
Pneumonia, 24, 33–36, 70, 103,
    129–130
Pneumothorax, 134
Pollen, 30, 60, 61
Polymask, 65
Postural drainage, 50, 71, 72, 93, 94
Prednisolone, 63
Pressure within pleural space, 12
Prevention of tuberculosis, 84
Primary bronchus, 4
Primary influenzal pneumonia, 41
Primary tuberculosis, 78, 81, 89
Promethazine, 64
Progressive massive fibrosis, 97
Protective reaction, 77
Prussic acid, 14
Psittacosis, 41, 43
Pulmonary embolism, 24
Pulmonary fibrosis, 95
Pulmonary infarction, 129
Pulmonary infiltration, 96
Pulmonary lesion, 78, 79
Pulsus alternans, 65
Purified protein derivative, 82
Pursing of lips, 24, 48
Pyopneumothorax, 135
Pyrazinamide, 88

Radioactive xenon, 19
Radiotherapy, 120
Residual air, 15
Respiration, 1, 9, 12
Respirometer, 55
Ribs, 1, 7, 9, 62, 121, 132
Rifampicin, 87

Saccular bronchiectasis, 89
Salbutamol, 53, 62
'Salvage drugs', 88
Sarcoidosis, 94
Scalene node biopsy, 96
Scoliosis, 28
Secondary tumours, 125
Segregation in tuberculosis, 85
Septicaemia, 43
Septrin, 42, 51
Serratus anterior muscle, 10
Shortness of breath, *see* Dyspnoea
Silicosis, 97

Silver nitrate, 137
Sinusitis, 67
Skin testing 66
Slow reacting substance, 60
Small intestine, ulceration of, 81
Smoking, 46, 53, 67, 99, 102
Sodium chromoglycate, 63
Spinal cord, 6, 72
Spirometer, 16
Spontaneous pneumothorax, 134
Sputum, 22, 31, 47, 50, 67, 68, 70, 71,
    75, 80, 81, 90, 92, 103, 106, 115
Squamous tumour, 101
Staphylococcal pneumonia, 35
Staphylococcus pyogenes, 35
Status asthmaticus, 61
Sternomastoid muscle, 10
Sternum, 5, 6, 12
Steroid drugs, 63
Stethoscope, 29
Streptomycin, 88
Sub phrenic abscess, 70, 131
Suffocation, 68
Sweating at night, 81
Symptoms of disease, 21

Temperature, 31, 35, 37, 41, 70, 131
Tension pneumothorax, 135, 136
Terbutaline, 62
Test for
    air exchange in alveoli, 19
    blood flow, 20
    coughing up blood, 23
    forced vital capacity, 17, 19
    nitrogen content of lungs, 19
    over-breathing, 14
    peak expiratory flow rate, 18
    skin condition, 65
    tubercle bacilli, 82
Tetany, 14
Thiotepa, 124
Thoracic aorta, 1
Thoracic breathing, 10
Thoracic cage, 5
Thoracic vertebrae, 6
Thoracoplasty, 89, 133
Thoracoscopy, 137
Thorax, 1–20
Thymus, 125
Tidal air, 16
Tiredness, 81
Tobacco, 99
Tomography, 109
Tongue, 3
Tonsil, 74
Trachea, 1, 2, 21, 68, 92
Tracheal intubation, 55, 64

Tracheobronchitis, 30
Tracheostomy, 55, 56, 64
Tracheal tube, 55
Tubercle bacilli, 74–80, 84, 85, 86
    isolation of 81
Tubercle of rib, 7
Tuberculin test, 83
Tuberculosis, 23, 77–80, 94, 129
    diagnosis, 85, 88
    infection, 75
    prevention, 84, 85
Tuberculous laryngitis, 81
Tuberculous lesions, 75, 78
Tuberculous meningitis, 80
Tubular bronchiectasis, 89
Tudor – Edwards spectacles, 52

Underwater drain, 113
Uraemia, 24, 139

Vagus nerve, 13
Valium, 42, 64
Vanishing lung, 48
Vascular system of thorax, 1

Ventilation, 15, 57–58, 64
Venti mask, 51, 65
Ventolin, 62, 63
Vertebral foramen, 6
Vinblastine, 124
Vincristine, 124
Viomycin, 88
Virus pneumonia, 40
Visceral pleura, 11, 133, 134
Vital capacity, 15
Vitalograph, 18
Vocal cords, 2
Voicebox, see Larynx
Vomiting of blood, see Haemoptysis

Wet pleurisy, 129–131
White blood cells, 34, 61, 131
Whooping cough, 90
Windpipe, see Trachea
Wright's peak flow meter, 18, 49

Xenon, 19
Xiphoid process, 6
Xylocaine, 109